THE POLITICS OF SICKLE CELL AND THALASSAEMIA

**Elizabeth N. Anionwu
and Karl Atkin**

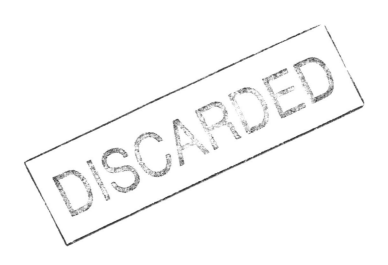

Open University Press
Buckingham · Philadelphia

Open University Press
Celtic Court
22 Ballmoor
Buckingham
MK18 1XW

email: enquiries@openup.co.uk
world wide web: www.openup.co.uk

and
325 Chestnut Street
Philadelphia, PA 19106, USA

First Published 2001

A catalogue record of this book is available from the British Library

ISBN   0 335 19607 1 (pb)   0 335 19608 X (hb)

Library of Congress Cataloging-in-Publication Data
Anionwu, Elizabeth N., 1947–
   The politics of sickle cell and thalassaemia / Elizabeth N. Anionwu and
   Karl Atkin.
       p.   cm. – (Race, health, and social care)
   Includes bibliographical references and index.
   ISBN 0-335-19608-X – ISBN 0-335-19607-1
   1. Sickle cell anemia–Political aspects.   2. Thalassaemia–Political
aspects.   I. Atkin, Karl.   II. Title.   III. Series.
RC641.7.S5 A54 2001
616.1'527–dc21
                                                                   00-050177

Typeset by Graphicraft Limited, Hong Kong
Printed in Great Britain by St Edmundsbury Press Ltd,
Bury St Edmunds, Suffolk

To my daughter Azuka, my mother Mrs Mary Hart and my late father, Mr Lawrence Odiatu Victor ('LOV') Anionwu (EA)

For Jane and Florence (KA)

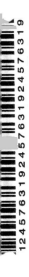

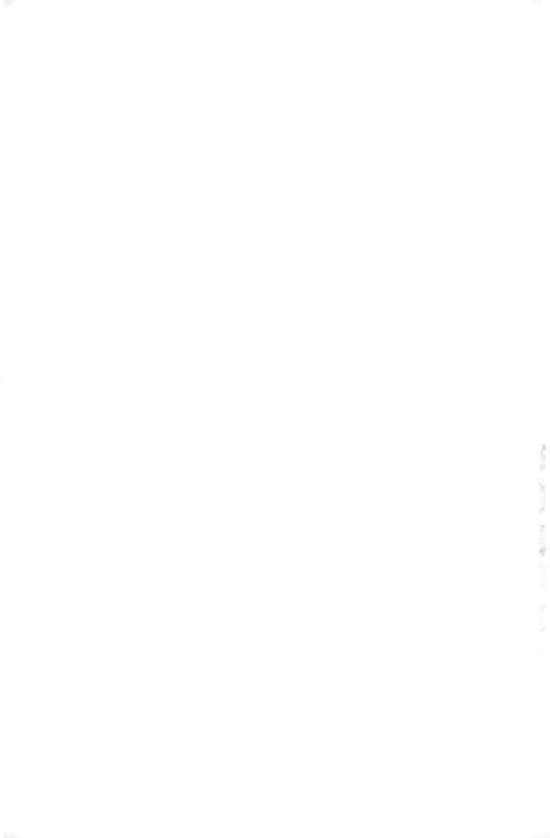

Contents

List of tables

Acknowledgements

Many people have contributed to this book. We are particularly indebted to all those affected by SCD and thalassaemia whom we know and have known, with special remembrance to those who are now deceased.

In addition, our thinking has also been informed by dialogue with members of voluntary community groups and haemoglobinopathy professionals. Inspiration and advice have been provided in a variety of ways and from a range of people, some for over a period of several decades. The support of individuals such as Dr Milica Brozovic, Alan Beattie, the late Professor Kermit Nash and Nina Patel date back to those early pioneering days of the late 1970s and early 1980s. In preparing this book we would especially like to thank Lorna Bennett, Deborah Collins, Dr Ade Olujohungbe, Professor Theresa Marteau, Dr Alison May, Professor Bernadette Modell, Professor Marcus Pembrey, Dr Anne Yardumian and staff of the NHS Executive Equal Opportunities Unit.

Waqar Ahmad provided helpful, supportive and constructive feedback throughout the production of the book. Hazel Blackburn helped considerably in producing the final manuscript. Finally we would like to thank Jacinta Evans and Clara Waissbein at Open University Press for their support and patience.

1

The politics of sickle cell disorders and thalassaemia

Government policy (Department of Health 1997) acknowledges the 'special health care needs' of UK's minority ethnic communities. Yet the two particular care needs of minority ethnic groups – sickle cell disorders (SCDs) and thalassaemia – have received little and belated recognition (Department of Health 1993; Health Education Authority 1998). The National Health Service has been slow to recognize haemoglobinopathies as significant public health issues (Anionwu 1996a). Those endeavouring to improve services, for example, have difficulties competing with the more 'traditional' concerns of an NHS, responding to the needs of a predominantly white population (Bradby 1996; Dyson 1998). Recognition among other sectors of welfare provision, such as social services, housing, social security and education, is even more limited (Ahmad and Atkin 1996a). Not only do local authorities have little understanding of haemoglobinopathies, they are also not especially interested in providing support to young people or families affected by the conditions (Atkin et al. 1998a). Social security officers regularly confuse SCDs (the condition) with sickle cell trait (carrier status) and benefits are often refused as a consequence of the assessors' ignorance (Atkin et al. 2000). Educational provision is similarly ill equipped to meet the needs of children and their families (Midence and Elander 1994; Atkin and Ahmad 2000a, 2000b).

Mistaken assumptions about the limited relevance of haemoglobinopathies to health and social care debates have helped keep them off the national social policy agenda, effectively stifling any chance of mainstream funds for development and research. There has been a reluctance to allocate regional or national funds for conditions that do not affect the majority population (Anionwu 1993). This is despite statistics questioning the myth that haemoglobinopathies are only relevant for a few urban conurbations (see Modell and Anionwu 1996; Hickman et al. 1999).

In the UK it is estimated that there are approximately 12,500 people with SCDs (Streetly et al. 1997) and over 700 people with thalassaemia major

(Modell *et al.* 2000b). The prevalence of these inherited blood disorders is greater than that for cystic fibrosis (Hodson 1989; Dodge *et al.* 1997) and haemophilia (Cowe 1995). The number of carriers is, of course, far larger. About 10 per cent of African-Caribbean people, for example, carry sickle cell trait, whereas 1 in 12 Pakistani people carry the thalassaemia trait (Modell and Anionwu 1996). Generally, the figures suggest that 6 per cent of the UK population and about 10 per cent of all births are in groups at risk for haemoglobinopathy disorders (Department of Health 1993). Hickman *et al.* (1999) have provided estimates of the prevalence of sickle cell and beta thalassaemia in England validated against six community screening programmes (see next chapter).

Arguments about numbers, however, often disguise a more fundamental reason for the neglect of haemoglobinopathies: their association with minority ethnic populations (Black and Laws 1986). Evidence suggests that British welfare services fail to adequately recognize and respond to the needs of people from minority ethnic groups (see Ahmad 1993; Ahmad and Atkin 1996a). Individual and institutional racism means the health and social care needs of minority ethnic groups are often neglected. This failure to acknowledge the existence of a multi-ethnic society has resulted in an inability to respond to haemoglobinopathies in an equitable and timely way (Anionwu 1993), and perhaps explains why community activists, even in metropolitan areas with the highest prevalence, have faced an uphill struggle to convince health authorities of the need for resources to develop provision (Atkin *et al.* 1998a, 1998b). An immediate response has been to marginalize the issue by denying mainstream monies while encouraging voluntary groups to apply for short-term grants (Department of Health 1993). This in itself is an example of institutional racism and does little to alter the response of mainstream agencies, while also leading to inadequate support for the populations concerned (Atkin 1996). More generally, racism can explain the low priority and poor coordination of haemoglobinopathy provision and professionals' negative attitudes (Atkin *et al.* 1998a, 1998b). Haemoglobinopathies, without much doubt, would have higher priority if they were not seen as 'black' conditions (Bradby 1996). This will become an important theme of the book.

Generally, sickle cell and thalassaemia provision have so far received relatively low priority and service development has occurred in response to public action rather than on the basis of routine assessment of population need (Anionwu 1993). Inadequate, ill coordinated and poorly resourced services present major problems for people with a haemoglobinopathy and their families alike (Department of Health 1993; Streetly *et al.* 1997; Health Education Authority 1998). Specific barriers to access include inadequate knowledge of conditions and limited information on the part of families and negative attitudes, as well as limited understanding among service practitioners (Darr 1990; Midence and Elander 1994; Atkin *et al.* 1998a; Atkin *et al.* 2000). Calls for better coordinated services both at a local as well as a national level have repeatedly been made by health workers (Davies *et al.*

1993; Streetly *et al.* 1997), patients' organizations (Sickle Cell Society 1981; Barnardo's 1993) and official working parties (Department of Health 1993; Health Education Authority 1998). As Franklin (1990: 86) notes:

> Services for sickle cell disease, although improving, are lagging behind the numbers of cases arising in the UK. Major obstacles to progress are the inadequate education of health professionals, disadvantage within the black community and institutionalised racism. It is unlikely that services will be improved unless there is a very vigorous and active co-operation between those providing services for patients and the self-help groups in lobbying budget holders and health care policy makers.

Franklin's comment regarding sickle cell disorders is equally applicable to thalassaemia.

Emancipation, empowerment and struggle

This book examines the politics of sickle cell and thalassaemia provision in the UK and is timely for a variety of reasons. In the first instance, after many years of neglect, there is increasing policy interest in haemoglobinopathies and how to improve existing provision (Department of Health 1993; Streetly *et al.* 1997; Health Education Authority 1998). This book will directly contribute to these debates and more generally, raise awareness of sickle cell and thalassaemia. In doing so, primacy will be accorded to patients' and their families' views. We will examine delivery and organization of services from users' perspectives. This fulfils another important aim of the book: to provide a detailed evaluation of UK haemoglobinopathy provision.

The book, however, is not just about haemoglobinopathies; it also addresses more general policy and practice interests. There is, for example, growing recognition of the care needs of minority ethnic groups and policy documents emphasize the need for a more systematic approach to planning and providing culturally sensitive services (Hopkins and Bahl 1993; Social Service Inspectorate 1994; Rawaf and Bahl 1998). Such initiatives occur against the backdrop of inaccessible and inappropriate provision (see Ahmad and Atkin 1996a). Haemoglobinopathy provision reflects many of the broader problems that deny minority ethnic communities adequate care and support. These include inadequate language support, inappropriate generalizations, poor quality of care as well as institutional and individual racism (Streetly *et al.* 1997; Atkin *et al.* 1998a, 1998b). To this extent, haemoglobinopathies represent a useful case study in examining the general difficulties faced by minority ethnic groups in having their needs recognized and met by welfare services (McNaught 1987).

More specifically, examples of good practice in haemoglobinopathy provision can inform improvements in more general provision to minority ethnic groups. Nor is this discussion simply about identifying examples of poor practice. The high regard in which families hold specialist haemo-globinopathy workers, for instance, reminds us that services for minority ethnic people can be sensitive and empowering (Atkin *et al.* 1998a). Another broad policy and practice theme concerns the increasing interest in the genetic basis of disease and the development of provision to identify such conditions (see Marteau and Richards 1996). Haemoglobinopathies are central to such debates (Atkin and Ahmad 1997). Sickle cell and thalas-saemia, for instance raise various issues at the heart of the 'new genetics' by illustrating the general complexities of screening and diagnosing reces-sive and other genetic disorders (Modell *et al.* 1998; Dyson 1999). As part of this debate, three significant themes emerge – explored more fully in Chapter 3. First, general practical problems include poor knowledge of the value and purpose of genetic screening among health professionals; late referral of women for prenatal diagnosis; the lack of coherent screening and counselling policy; and poor interagency collaboration (compare Green and Murton 1996; Atkin *et al.* 1998b; Modell *et al.* 2000a). Second, screen-ing and counselling provision implicates more philosophical concerns such as the tension between 'informed decision making' and 'prevention' (Atkin and Ahmad 1997). Third, evidence suggests a mismatch between profes-sional and lay logic regarding genetics (Richards and Green 1993; Atkin *et al.* 1998b). Individuals do not make simple choices in light of relevant information; a variety of personal and social factors influence their decisions (Michie and Marteau 1996).

Besides its contribution to debates about the 'new genetics', this book will also add to our general understanding of chronic illness and family caregiving among minority ethnic groups. These are much-neglected areas in sociology and social policy, which itself is perhaps a reflection of the institutionalized nature of British racism (Ahmad 1993). We know little about the organization and experience of family caregiving among minority ethnic groups (Atkin and Rollings 1996). There is even less material addressing the experiences of and disadvantages associated with, disability and chronic illness (Stuart 1996). The emerging literature on sickle cell and thalassaemia – when linked to other material – can help make sense of the experience of chronic illness for minority ethnic people as well as the organization of family care.

Finally, empowerment and struggle in improving the lives of minority ethnic communities becomes a fundamental unifying theme informing our narrative. Many of the improvements in the provision of sickle cell and thalassaemia services have occurred as a consequence of community action (Atkin *et al.* 1998b). This reminds us of the importance of informed eman-cipatory struggle grounded in critical analysis (see Gramsci 1957) and active citizenship (Held 1989). The continuing strategy and struggle faced by minority ethnic groups in ensuring that sickle cell and thalassaemia gain recognition by mainstream agencies provides useful insights into the pol-itics of 'race'. Writings on 'race' and welfare provision tend to focus on the unfair structuring of opportunities (Atkin and Rollings 1993). The critical emphasis of the literature is perhaps understandable and has successfully highlighted the negative consequences of racism, marginalization and unequal treatment (see Ahmad 1993). Nonetheless by focusing on disadvantage there is a danger of adopting a 'victim orientated' perspective that undervalues the significance and contributions of the struggle of 'black' led organizations. Maulana Karenga described the dilemma:

> How does one prove strength in opposition without overstating the case? Diluting criticisms of the system and absolving the oppressor in the process? How does one criticise the system and state of things without contributing to the victimology school which thrives on litanies of lost battles and casualty lists, while omitting victories and strengths and the possibilities for change inherent in both black people and society.
>
> (cited in Jeyasingham 1992: 1)

Constantly highlighting the negative consequences of service provision does little to advance thinking and practice (Levick 1992). Therefore, accounts acknowledging the significance and success of struggles to improve conditions need to supplement work stressing the negative consequences of racism in welfare provision.

Following this, focusing on the needs of minority ethnic groups is not the same as meeting those needs. Action is required. The disadvantages experienced by minority ethnic groups are not inevitable. Despite the overwhelming power of established institutions in Britain, there is frequently scope for successful pressure from the grass roots (Farrah 1986). Policy and practice are made up of contradictory and changeable elements that create 'radical possibilities' (Harrison 1993). Haemoglobinopathy provision in the UK represents a particularly good case study highlighting both the threats and opportunities faced by minority ethnic communities. Despite a constraining and sometimes hostile external environment, community action on haemoglobinopathies offers an example of positive achievement and is a reminder of what struggle and emancipatory activity can accomplish. The emergence of such community action demonstrates that resistance, dissent and grass-roots pressure can empower people from ethnic minorities. In effect, minority ethnic people have to be aware of their rights and the value of taking subsequent action to secure them. The emergence of national and local voluntary organizations in sickle cell and thalassaemia reflects the potential of empowerment and struggle by focusing on strategies, resources and forms of support that African-Caribbean and South Asian people find helpful.

Locating the book in wider discussions about social policy further contributes to this strategy and struggle, by suggesting possible alliances with other disadvantaged groups. Debates about haemoglobinopathies are typically marginalized and divorced from the mainstream concerns of social policy and political philosophy. It is possible for example, to compare the experience of parents who care for a child with a haemoglobinopathy and those who care for children with other chronic illnesses (Thompson 1994a, 1994b). Many of the difficulties they face are alike. Their views on accessible and appropriate provision also have similarities (see Ahmad and Atkin, 1996b; Beresford 1996a, 1996b). Screening and counselling for haemoglobin-opathies also raises generic problems, faced by those at risk of recessive disorders as well as those providing support. More generally – as we shall see in Chapter 4 – those with a haemoglobinopathy also face many of the disadvantages and discrimination experienced by disabled and chronically ill people in general. Consequently, there are possible links between differ-ent groups aimed at improving general service provision rather than piece-meal battles that make limited advances, often only improving the position of small, narrowly defined groups. This is an issue we address throughout the book.

Structure of the book

The book's structure reflects the broad policy themes described above. At its most straightforward, it offers an introduction to haemoglobinopathies. The book will also address more general policy concerns. As we have seen, these include examining the general difficulties of providing accessible and appropriate welfare support as well as engaging with more specific debates about the 'new genetics' and the experience of chronic illness and family caregiving among minority ethnic communities. Perhaps more importantly, however, the book provides an account of struggle, emphasizing its import-ance in gaining recognition of the needs of minority ethnic groups. Not only is this a central theme of the book, but in turn, the book hopes to make a contribution to these debates by providing a critical analysis aimed at ensuring haemoglobinopathies receive the attention and support they deserve.

Following this brief introduction, Chapters 2 and 3 provide a clinical introduction to haemoglobinopathies. This clinical description examines the origins of sickle cell and thalassaemia as well as their incidence, identi-fication and consequences. The two chapters aim to present a detailed account of haemoglobinopathies. This is particularly important because the limited understanding of sickle cell or thalassaemia held by many prac-titioners and managers results in inadequate care and support for affected individuals and their families (Atkin *et al.* 1998a). The description of haemoglobinopathies will also provide the broader context for the remainder of the book and will allow the reader to make sense of the text. Acknow-ledging these clinical influences, however, is not intended to support a med-ical model of disability. There is a long-standing critique of the medical model of disability, suggesting that an overemphasis on medical concerns marginalizes an individual's experience of their condition and ignores the way in which the disadvantages they face have social and material causes (Oliver 1996). This book generally accepts this critique and will illustrate its value when discussing haemoglobinopathies. This is a particular feature of Chapter 4 and as we shall see, those with the illness can find themselves excluded from certain types of social, political and economic activity because of the inflexible attitudes of the wider society. Nonetheless it is also important to accept that the experience of chronic illness cannot fully transcend the origins or consequences of the initial impairment (Morris 1991).

Chapter 4 explores screening and diagnosing within the context of the 'new genetics'. It begins by examining some of the ethical dilemmas in screening and diagnosing haemoglobinopathies, before considering the problems of establishing and managing an accessible and appropriate service. In doing so, it identifies specific shortfalls in current provision and provides philosophical and practical insights into how they can be addressed.

Chapter 5 outlines the general problems faced by those with the illness and their families, as well as the strategies they adopt to cope with their illness on a daily basis. This is not intended to offer a straightforward narrative outlining the relevant literature. This can be found elsewhere (see Midence and Elander 1994). The purpose is to provide an insight into living with a haemoglobinopathy within the broader social context. Such a discussion begins to identify legitimate areas of strategy and struggle, aimed at improving understanding and support for those with the illness and their families. The chapter also draws out similarities with other disadvantaged groups and thereby suggests possible alliances.

Chapter 6 examines present shortfalls in provision, before focusing on examples of good practice which adds to our understanding. For example, rectifying shortfalls in provision as well as building on existing good practice, suggests a possible agenda for community action as well as state intervention. Chapter 6 also reminds us how haemoglobinopathy provision is thus caught up in the general struggle for more equitable provision faced by minority ethnic groups.

The final chapter considers the historical development of haemoglobinopathy services in the UK, bringing out the importance of strategy and struggle. It ends by looking towards the future by identifying both opportunities and threats, while also arguing that haemoglobinopathy services can build on the successes of the past 20 years.

2

Origins, geographic distribution, genetics and laboratory investigations

The figures suggest that about six per cent of the population of England and about ten per cent of all births are in groups at risk for haemoglobinopathy disorders. Though ethnic minorities tend to be concentrated in the conurbations, every NHS Region has at least one area with a significant number of births in relevant ethnic groups.

(Department of Health 1993: 15)

In Chapters 2 and 3 we provide an introduction to sickle cell and thalassaemia disorders. This is an important starting point, because as we have argued in the previous chapter, lack of understanding about these conditions results in a major form of disadvantage facing minority ethnic groups. The two chapters also provide a broader context for the rest of the book by setting out the historical milestones as well as current knowledge about the origins, natural history and management of the two disorders. We will begin our account with a discussion about the origins of sickle cell and thalassaemia.

Origins and current geographic distribution of sickle cell and thalassaemia

There are various types of sickle cell and thalassaemia disorders, also known as haemoglobinopathies or haemoglobin (Hb) disorders. The thalassaemia syndromes include alpha and beta thalassaemia major as well as beta thalassaemia intermedia. Sickle cell disorders (or sickle cell disease) include sickle cell anaemia (Hb SS), sickle haemoglobin C disease (Hb SC) and sickle beta thalassaemia. Thalassaemia syndromes include Hb H disease and E beta thalassaemia. Table 2.1 provides a more detailed list.

Sickle cell and thalassaemia disorders mainly affect individuals who are descended from families where one or more members originated from parts

Table 2.1 The most common types of sickle cell and thalassaemia disorders seen in the UK

Sickle cell disorders	Thalassaemia syndromes
• Sickle cell anaemia (Hb SS) • Sickle beta thalassaemia • Hb SC disease • Hb SD disease • Hb SE disease • Other rare sickle cell disorders	• Beta thalassaemia major • Beta thalassaemia intermedia • Hb E beta thalassaemia • Other rare forms of thalassaemia • Alpha thalassaemia major (Hb Barts hydrops fetalis) • Hb H disease

Source: adapted from Department of Health 1993

of the world where falciparum malaria was, or is still, endemic. Populations with such ancestry include those from many parts of Africa, the Caribbean, the Mediterranean (including southern Italy, northern Greece and southern Turkey), Southeast Asia, and the Middle and Far East (Serjeant 1992: 23). The distribution of the sickle and thalassaemia gene is much wider now due to the historical movements of at-risk populations to North and South America, the Caribbean and Western Europe (Livingstone 1985).

Nagel (1994) has produced a comprehensive review of the origin and dispersion of the sickle gene and this provides an interesting case study in how racist myths, rather than scientific insight, drive debates. The more recent introduction of universal screening programmes, where people are tested regardless of ethnic origin, suggests that the sickle gene is found in many ethnic groups. This counters the myth that sickle cell is a 'black' disease. US neonatal screening programmes, for example, have noted mean prevalence rates per 100,000 populations of sickle cell trait in whites to be between 242 to 258 and for sickle cell disease, to be between 1.72 and 1.90 (Sickle Cell Disease Guideline Panel 1993). A study of parents of newborns identified with sickle cell trait through a neonatal screening programme in Rochester, New York, noted that, 'Not all individuals with sickle cell trait are black. In this group, eleven per cent were Hispanic, Italian, or of other ethnic groups, some of whom were surprised to learn that they carry a sickle gene' (Rowley 1989: 891). There have been similar findings in Florida with Mack (1989: 862) commenting that, 'The common belief that they [Hb S and Hb C] occur only in blacks results in a reluctance to consider the diagnosis or to accept it when made, because to do so implies racial intermixing.' As Powars concludes (1994a: 1885) 'Today, patients with sickle cell disease (SCD) range from individuals with blond hair and blue eyes to those with olive skin and straight dark hair to those with dark skin and curly black hair.' She also highlights that in urban centres in the United States nearly 10 per cent of patients with various sickling disorders identify themselves as non-black. There remain those, however, who could not accept the diagnosis of sickle cell disorders in 'non-blacks'. As Tapper (1999: 28) notes:

> In the first half of the twentieth century, 'sickling' played an important role in substantiating the notion of the racial distinctiveness of 'white' and 'black' bodies and, paradoxically, in destabilising the very notion of whiteness: Sometimes a Caucasian is not a Caucasian . . . It is ironic that this destabilisation of whiteness would take place in the work of physicians who thought themselves as attending to the science or truth of the black body and its signs.

Such misconceptions still occur despite the increasing recognition that the sickle cell gene is found in white populations (Gelpi and Perrine 1973; Serjeant 1992) and this often confuses the debate about screening (Atkin *et al*. 1998b and see Chapter 4).

Malaria and haemoglobin disorders

The original occurrence of haemoglobin disorders in areas where malaria is found suggested a possible connection and we now know that the healthy carrier-state (also known as a trait) appears to offer some protection in early childhood against malaria. The highest gene frequencies for sickle haemoglobin, for example, occur in the so-called 'malarial belt' of Equatorial Africa – where the prevalence of the sickle gene ranges from 1 to 45 per cent of the population (Serjeant 1992). Allison (1957), building on Neel's (1947) earlier work, was the first to propose that the sickle cell gene may have an evolutionary value, with the carrier (heterozygote) having a special advantage not enjoyed by either those with the illness (such as Hb SS) or the usual haemoglobin type (Hb AA). His studies in Kenya demonstrated that a carrier for sickle haemoglobin had an increased resistance to falciparum malaria. Other likely examples where similar protection is thought to be afforded include carriers for haemoglobins C, E and the thalassaemias (Eaton 1994).

   Racist myths, however, again hindered this understanding and meant the link between malaria and the origins of the sickle gene were not accepted in all quarters (Tapper 1999). Until the 1950s, for example, medical discourse was confused over the higher prevalence of sickle cell trait and apparent lack of cases of sickle cell anaemia in certain parts of Africa compared to the situation in the United States. People had failed to realize, however, that the lack of cases in Africa was due to the high death rates of infants with sickle cell disorders, mainly due to malaria. One alternate and popular suggestion to account for the link was that, compared to those people in Africa, the blood of African-Americans was now being diluted with white blood. Tapper (1999), for instance, cites Ashman (1952) who argued 'that the disease originated as a by-product of racial mixture' rather than recessive genes.

Such myths set back our understanding of haemoglobin disorders by many years and especially confused our understanding of the genetic basis of haemoglobin disorders. Despite work in the 1920s and 1930s suggesting a possible genetic link, it was not until the early 1950s that this became commonly understood. Serjeant (1992) provides the most useful historical review of sickle cell trait and suggests that initial recognition of sickle cell trait occurred in the 1920s (see Huck 1923; Sydenstricker 1924). Diggs *et al.* (1933), however, first clearly distinguished between cases with symptoms, which they called *sickle cell anaemia* from those without, for which they proposed the term *sickle cell trait*. Fifteen years later Neel (1947) was among the first to suggest the recessive mode of inheritance for sickle cell disorders in studies that set out to explain the difference between the asymptomatic parents and their children with symptoms of sickle cell anaemia. Beet (1949) provided further evidence in one large family study undertaken in Zambia which showed the inherited nature of sickle cell anaemia while Neel (1949) reported similar findings from 29 families in the United States of America. The development of haemoglobin electrophoresis in the 1950s (to be described later in the chapter) confirmed beyond doubt the differentiation between sickle cell anaemia (Hb SS) and sickle cell trait (Hb AS).

This distinction contributed directly to understanding the molecular basis of haemoglobin disorders, which were among the first to be recognized as molecular diseases. As long ago as 1949 Linus Pauling, a noted American physical chemist, established the molecular basis of sickle cell anaemia (Pauling *et al.* 1949). Strasser (1999: 1490) argues Pauling's legacy should not be underestimated:

> Pauling's grand vision of molecular biology and medicine has been realised to an extent he could never have foreseen, even if our therapeutic power does not yet match our understanding of the molecular basis of disease.

Haemoglobin, the oxygen-carrying protein in red blood cells, is comprised of alpha and beta globin chains. Sickle cell disorders result from a problem with the *quality* of the beta globin chains rather than the quantity. Thalassaemias, on the other hand, are due to a partial or total reduction in the *quantity* of either the alpha or beta globin chains. The exact location of the alpha and beta globin genes have been known for some time – the alpha globin gene on chromosome 16 (Deisseroth *et al.* 1977) and the beta globin gene on chromosome 11 (Deisseroth *et al.* 1978). Beta globin chains are proteins set out in an orderly sequence of 146 amino acids. The structure of sickle beta haemoglobin (also known as Beta^S or Hb S) differs to that of adult haemoglobin (Beta^A or Hb A) by just one alteration in the amino acid sequence on the beta globin chain. Glutamic acid is the sixth amino acid in the beta globin sub-unit of adult haemoglobin (Beta^A) whereas in sickle haemoglobin (Beta^S) it has been replaced by valine. In haemoglobin C (Beta^C) there is also an alteration of the sixth amino acid, with glutamic acid now replaced by lysine.

Inheritance of sickle cell and thalassaemia disorders

The recessive inheritance of haemoglobin disorders, despite initial scepticism, is now fully established. The illnesses, equally distributed between boys and girls, are inherited from both parents who are generally healthy carriers of a trait such as beta thalassaemia or sickle cell trait. It has been estimated that, depending upon ethnic group, there will be 17–100 times as many healthy carriers as affected children. The frequencies of the different traits for haemoglobinopathies in various ethnic groups are shown in Table 2.2.

Where a couple are both healthy carriers of a trait there is, in every pregnancy, a 25 per cent chance of having a child with a sickle cell or thalassaemia disorder, a 25 per cent chance of having one with the usual haemoglobin type and a 50 per cent chance that the child will inherit the trait. This is often communicated as a 1 in 4 chance of having children with the illness but it needs to be stressed that this chance applies to *each and every pregnancy*. Otherwise at-risk couples may believe that if they already have one child with the illness, the next three will not (see Chapter 4). Equally it is possible for parents who both carry a trait to have no affected children whatsoever.

Table 2.2   Examples of some carrier frequencies of haemoglobinopathies in various ethnic groups

Haemoglobin type	Ethnic group	Estimated carrier frequency
Beta thalassaemia trait	Cypriots	1 in 7
	Asians	1 in 10–30
	Chinese	1 in 30
	Afro-Caribbeans	1 in 50
	White British	1 in 1000
Alpha zero thalassaemia trait	Chinese	1 in 15–30
	Cypriots	1 in 50–100
Sickle cell trait	Afro-Caribbeans	1 in 10
	West Africans	1 in 4
	Cypriots	1 in 100
	Pakistanis, Indians	1 in 100
C trait	Afro-Caribbeans	1 in 30
	Ghanaians	up to 1 in 6
D trait	Pakistanis, Indians	1 in 100
	White British	1 in 1000

NB: The above does not include all ethnic groups at risk of haemoglobinopathies.
Source: Department of Health 1993

Sickle cell and thalassaemia traits are not illnesses and must always be distinguished from the disorders they cause. We explore the importance of maintaining this distinction in the next chapter. Sickle cell trait occurs when one parent passes on a gene for sickle haemoglobin and the other parent a gene for the usual haemoglobin. A person with sickle cell trait has more normal haemoglobin than sickle haemoglobin within each red blood cell. Consequently, 'sickling' of the red blood cells and associated problems are extremely rare occurrences (Serjeant 1992; Sears 1994). Research has provided findings that both confirms this (Heller *et al.* 1979; Hoiberg *et al.* 1981) as well as clarifying the type of complications that can occur (Kark *et al.* 1987). A major study by Heller *et al.* (1979) failed to demonstrate any difference in the age, duration, or the pattern of hospital admissions in black males with sickle cell trait compared to normal controls, a finding repeated by Hoiberg *et al.* (1981). However in a study by Kark *et al.* (1987) of all natural deaths of United States Armed Forces recruits between 1977 and 1981 – a total of 62 – it was noted that all of the 12 cases of sudden unexplained death in subjects with AS haemoglobin occurred during exertion. Such cases, although occurring in just less than 1 in 3000 black male army recruits, represented a 28-fold increase in risk compared to blacks with the normal haemoglobin type. Sears (1994) has summarized the main risks, that while rare, are associated with sickle cell trait. They include spleen complications at high altitude (splenic infarct), blood in the urine (haematuria), urine and kidney infections in pregnancy, sudden death following exertion, and clotting in the lung (pulmonary embolism). It does need to be emphasized, however, that the vast majority of individuals with sickle cell trait are perfectly healthy and will never be aware of their status unless they have their blood tested. The significant genetic information for individuals with sickle cell trait is that they are at risk of having children with a sickle cell disorder should their partner also have a trait or a disorder (see Chapter 4).

Thalassaemia trait is transmitted in the same way as sickle cell trait. In addition to the previously mentioned advantage that thalassaemia trait carriers have in respect to falciparum malaria the hypothesis that it may also provide some protection against heart attacks, otherwise known as a myocardial infarction (Crowley *et al.* 1987) appears to have been confirmed (Wang and Schilling 1995). Ironically, as the blood picture of beta thalassaemia trait resembles that of iron-deficiency anaemia, there has been a history of healthy carriers being unnecessarily treated with iron supplements (Modell and Berdoukas 1984). As with SCD, the trait should not be regarded as an illness.

Frequency of sickle cell and thalassaemia disorders and traits

The haemoglobinopathies account for some of the most common single gene disorders in the world (Weatherall 1999), with at least 5 per cent of the world's population being carriers for one or other of the most serious types. Worldwide estimates for the number of those with a haemoglobin disorder vary. Angastiniotis and Modell (1998) suggest that over 300,000 infants are born each year with the major sickle cell and thalassaemia syndromes and that the majority die undiagnosed, untreated or undertreated. Serjeant (1997) estimates that 250,000 children are born with sickle cell disorders worldwide and Steinberg (1999) notes that 120,000 such babies are born in Africa each year compared to 1,000 in the United States. Weatherall (1996) has provided illustrations to justify that thalassaemia syndromes (particularly the beta thalassaemias and haemoglobin E/beta thalassaemia) are a global public health problem. In parts of the world such as the Middle East, the Indian subcontinent and Southeast Asia, thousands of children with beta thalassaemia major are born annually. He notes that over the next 30 years approximately 100,000 new cases of haemoglobin E thalassaemia alone (a disorder that produces a very severe form of anaemia) will be added to the population.

Hickman *et al.* (1999) have calculated that annually in England approximately 3000 babies (0.47 per cent) are born with sickle cell trait and 2800 (0.44 per cent) carry beta thalassaemia trait. Approximately 178 (0.28 per 1000 conception) are affected with sickle cell disorders and 43 (0.07 per 1000) with beta thalassaemia major or intermedia. When termination is taken into account, about 140–75 babies affected with SCD and 10–25 with beta thalassaemia major/intermedia are born annually in England. The data indicates that, although the greatest proportion (45 per cent) of affected populations live in a limited number of 'high prevalence' district health authorities with more than 20 per cent of minority ethnic residents, 35 per cent live in district health authorities where ethnic minority population accounts for 5–20 per cent of the total population. Moreover, over 20 per cent live in 'low prevalence' areas with less than 5 per cent minority ethnic populations (Modell and Anionwu 1996).

Laboratory investigations

Haemoglobinopathy screening entails a variety of laboratory tests in order to detect the different forms of sickle cell disorders, thalassaemias and their carrier states, in both the adult, the newborn and the unborn fetus (British Committee for Standards in Haematology 1994; Zeuner *et al.* 1999; Davies *et al.* 2000). Table 2.3 details laboratory investigations that can be used for haemoglobinopathy screening and diagnosis. Broadly speaking, laboratory investigations for the diagnosis of haemoglobinopathies need to be precise and comprehensive. A golden rule for anybody involved with genetic counselling is to ensure that, before the session starts, they obtain a written copy of the laboratory results.

Table 2.3 Laboratory investigations that can be used for haemoglobinopathy screening and diagnosis

A full blood count	This is an initial automated analysis of the blood sample that will include measurement of various red cell indices including the haemoglobin level for evidence of anaemia. In addition the size of the red blood cells will be measured and, if they are small (microcytic), could indicate a thalassaemia trait and/or iron deficiency. Investigations that can help to establish whether a person is a carrier for beta thalassaemia include the measurement of Hb A_2 (we discuss this below). Assessment of iron levels (e.g. serum ferritin) may also be required, particularly in pregnancy.
Haemoglobin electrophoresis	This technique separates different haemoglobins present in haemoglobin on the basis of their electrical charge when in a solution on a medium such as cellulose acetate or citrate agar. Hb S, F and A move faster and are further from the origin whereas Hb C moves slowly and is closest to the origin. This technique can thus help to distinguish between sickle cell anaemia (Hb SS), haemoglobin SC disease and the carrier states such as sickle cell trait (Hb AS) or C trait (Hb AC). However some haemoglobins move at the same rate on cellulose acetate and examples include Hb S and Hb D Punjab and Hb C and Hb O Arab. Other supplementary methods are therefore required for differentiation such as haemoglobin electrophoresis at different pH using citrate agar gel. In addition other diagnostic techniques, such as the sickling or solubility test, are also used. A sample that appears to have a band at Hb S (on a cellulose acetate electrophoresis) but has a sickle negative result may then be identified as Hb D Punjab using citrate agar haemoglobin electrophoresis. Other haemoglobin electrophoretic methods include: • Isoelectric focusing: This is a more expensive method but with higher resolution that has been found helpful in neonatal screening programmes (Galacteros *et al*. 1980). • High-Performance Liquid Chromatography (HPLC): HPLC is an automated method of separating haemoglobins (Wilson *et al*. 1983; Samperi *et al*. 1991; Lorey *et al*. 1994) and has

Table 2.3   (cont'd)

	been recommended for use in haemoglobinopathy screening, particularly at a regional level (International Committee for Standardization for Haemoglobinopathies 1988).
Sickle/Solubility tests	There are a variety of tests available that detect uniquely for the presence or absence of sickle haemoglobin. False negatives can occur if the solution becomes stale or in the neonatal period because the level of Hb S is insufficient to deform the cells. It is therefore a test that should not be used in testing newborn babies where the majority of haemoglobin is Hb F even if the child has Hb SS and should never be used as a primary screen test for anybody (J.G. Adams 1994).
Quantitation of haemoglobin A₂ and F	Ascertaining the amount of Hb A_2 is important as a diagnostic test for beta thalassaemia trait as it is usually raised to between 3.5 and 7 per cent in carriers (British Committee for Standards in Haematology 1994; *Journal of Medical Screening* 1998). A higher than average level of fetal haemoglobin (Hb F) may be present in beta thalassaemia, and very high levels could indicate hereditary persistence of fetal haemoglobin syndromes. A high level of Hb F in association with sickle cell anaemia may result in a very mild clinical course.
DNA analysis	An array of genetic technology such as restriction enzymes, DNA polymerase and DNA probes now facilitate detection of the haemoglobin genotype of the unborn baby (Globin Gene Disorder Working Party 1994; World Health Organization 1994). Cells from the chorionic villus or amniotic fluid can be multiplied using the polymerase chain reaction (PCR) technique. This, together with the use of DNA probes and other genetic technology (Old 1996), allows the identification of deletions and mutations on chromosomes 11 (for the beta globin gene) and 16 (for the alpha globin gene).

Prenatal diagnosis

Prenatal diagnosis is offered to couples at risk of having a child with a major haemoglobinopathy, that is if both are carriers or themselves have a sickle cell or thalassaemia disorder. There are three methods that can be used in pregnancy to test whether the unborn baby has inherited sickle cell or thalassaemia disorders (Royal College of Physicians 1989; Brock *et al.* 1992). All these techniques require ultrasound guidance and each carries a particular risk of miscarriage. This risk depends both upon the actual technique and the experience of the operator.

First, chorionic villus sampling (CVS) can be undertaken in the first trimester (Old *et al.* 1982, 1986; Petrou *et al.* 1983) with the best timing now thought to be sometime after the tenth week of pregnancy. This is in order to reduce the risk of limb abnormalities that may occur with early CVS (Evans and Hamerton 1996). It involves obtaining a sample of the chorionic villus, the tissue that surrounds the fetus and which later develops into the placenta (Silverman and Wapner 1992). Genetic investigations, such as DNA analysis, can then be carried out on the chorionic villus sample as it contains the genetic material that the fetus has inherited from the parents. The risk of miscarriage may range from 2 to 4 per cent (Royal College of Physicians 1989).

Amniocentesis is the second method. The fluid surrounding the unborn baby (amniotic fluid) also contains fetal cells that can be cultured and analysed to obtain genetic information and it has traditionally been carried out from week 16 of pregnancy (Kan and Dozy 1978; Maclachlan 1992). The risk of miscarriage ranges from 1 to 2 per cent (Royal College of Physicians 1989). Results may take longer to obtain than with CVS as it can take at least a week to grow the amniotic cells in culture.

Third, there is fetal blood sampling. When DNA diagnosis for haemoglobinopathies is not possible, blood can be obtained from the fetal cord of the unborn baby at approximately 17–18 weeks gestation (Kan *et al.* 1972). The risk of miscarriage, at around 5 per cent, is higher than with CVS or amniocentesis. The fetal blood sample can be analysed using techniques such as globin chain synthesis. Haemoglobinopathies were the first disorders to be diagnosed prenatally using this type of advanced DNA technology (Weatherall 1996).

These developments in screening and diagnosis for sickle cell and thalassaemia still leave a dilemma for those at-risk couples offered it as they have to determine the severity of the disorders with which their children may be born. The complexity of this is set out in the next chapter that describes the varied clinical features, management and likelihood of survival for each disorder.

Conclusion

This chapter is the first of two that present the more clinical aspects of haemoglobinopathies. This provides an important introduction to the book, particularly since a lack of understanding about sickle cell and thalassaemia creates major disadvantages for minority ethnic communities. Our discussion has also begun to identify other themes central to our account, such as how racism can influence supposed 'scientific' debates. The next chapter explores these issues further by discussing the clinical consequences of haemoglobinopathies.

3

Clinical features and management

This chapter charts some of the key historical developments that have led to our current understanding of the problems and management of sickle cell and thalassaemia disorders. In doing so we will also explore gaps in this understanding together with contemporary debates and conflicts surrounding treatment, attitudes of professionals and possible therapies for the future.

Sickle cell disorders

Historical milestones in the identification of sickle cell disorders

Herrick (1910) first used the term 'sickle' in an article describing the shape of the red blood cells of a 20-year-old student from Grenada. The patient first consulted him in 1904 complaining of a cough, fever and feeling weak and dizzy. He had repeated episodes of anaemia, jaundice, chest complications as well as recurring leg ulcers on both ankles. Examination of the red blood cells showed a 'large number of thin, elongated, sickle shaped and crescent-shaped forms' (Herrick 1910: 519). The fate of this patient, Walter Clement Noel, has been described by Savitt and Goldberg (1989). He came from a wealthy land-owning family in Grenada and studied dentistry in Chicago. After graduating in 1907 he returned to Grenada and set up a private dental practice in the capital, St Georges. At the age of 32 he developed pneumonia and died in May 1916; a photograph of his grave is featured in Serjeant's book (1992). It took, however, many more years before the inheritance, complications and treatment of sickle cell disorders were fully recognized (see previous chapter). We can only surmise at the historical impact that the ignorance surrounding this condition had on the care and chance of survival of affected individuals (Tapper 1999).

There is evidence, however, that West African people have been conversant with the clinical problems associated with sickle cell disorders for many centuries (Konotey-Ahulu 1968, 1974). There are, for example, several tribal vernacular names given to reflect the relentless and frequent episodes of bone pain such as chwechweechwe (Ga) and nwiiwii (Fanta). In addition one family belonging to the Krobo tribe in Ghana described the condition so accurately that Konotey-Ahulu was able to trace SCD in nine genera- tions, dating back to 1670 (Konotey-Ahulu 1974). Africanus Horton (1874) has been attributed with the first recorded description in Africa, when he described the fever of crises, the shifting joint pains, the exacerbation during the rainy season, and the constant abnormality of the blood.

The genetic basis of the illness may well be reflected in certain traditional health beliefs concerning reincarnation. Edelstein (1986) has described the role of the hierarchy of supernatural entities and cited a study of the death concepts of the Igbos in eastern Nigeria. Seven causes of death are listed, one of which was limited to children who were called 'ogbanje', meaning children who come and go or 'repeater children'. Similar terms of rein- carnation are found in other parts of the country such as 'àbikú' among the Yoruba people from southwest Nigeria and 'ekabasi' among the Efiks in southern Nigeria. In his study Edelstein found that these terms were not exclusively used for those who have died due to sickle cell anaemia, rather for when several young children die in a family, regardless of the possible cause.

Serjeant (1992) also describes two case reports prior to Herrick, that are suggestive of sickle cell disorders. The first by Lebby (1846) records the results of an autopsy he performed on a runaway slave executed for murder. Previous history included a full chest, narrow build and intermittent and remittent fevers. At autopsy the 'spleen was wanting'. The second case, reported by Hodenpyl in 1898, featured a 32-year-old black male who presented with generalized pain, chest symptoms, jaundice and was noted to have scars on the anterior surfaces of both legs. He died in hospital and no evidence of a spleen could be found at autopsy.

Numerous historical reviews (Conley 1980; Bessis and Delpech 1982; Fleming 1982; Serjeant 1992; Ranney 1994) have charted the developments since Herrick's paper. By 1922 a total of four cases had been described in the American medical literature including the original case reported by Herrick (1910). The second account was provided by Washburn (1911) of Virginia who wrote about a 25-year-old black woman whose main complaints were weakness, breathlessness, episodes of pain, swelling of the wrists and ankles, and leg ulcerations. She had had gallstones (a possible clinical feature of SCD) removed at the age of 23. Another case was re- ported from St Louis (Cook and Meyer 1915) and referred to a 21-year-old mulatto woman with a history of rheumatism, leg ulceration and severe anaemia. She was pale, jaundiced, and had a large heart with a systolic murmur. Her family were investigated by Emmel, Professor of Anatomy in Chicago, who had an interest in this condition. He noted the familial nature of the disease and suggested that sickling of the red blood cells might be linked to diminished oxygen supply (Emmel 1917). The fourth case, reported by Mason (1922: 1320) in Los Angeles, included the term anaemia, and he commented that:

> The blood picture does not resemble that seen in any of the more common anemias, and it is possible that the disease represents a clinical entity. If that is true, it is a particular interest that up to the present the malady has been seen only in the negro and, so far as could be ascertained, it is the only disease peculiar to that race.

Types of sickle cell disorders

We now know more about the origins and prognosis of sickle cell and provide an account of the main types of SCDs and the main complications associated with them. As we have seen, there are many types of sickle cell disorders (SCD) of which sickle cell anaemia is generally the commonest and most severe (Serjeant 1992). In the early 1950s, other types of sickle cell disorders were recognized. Examples included sickle beta thalassaemia (e.g. Powell *et al.* 1950; Silvestroni and Bianco 1952), haemoglobin SC disease (Kaplan *et al.* 1951; Neel *et al.* 1953) and SD Punjab (Sturgeon *et al.* 1955). Other types comprise SE and SO Arab disease. We now discuss these different variations in more detail. Healthy carrier states such as sickle cell trait are not, however, included in our discussion of sickle cell disorders (see previous chapter) nor combinations of variant haemoglobin genotypes that do not contain sickle haemoglobin – examples include CC, DD or EE.

Sickle cell anaemia
The incidence of children born with sickle cell anaemia (Haemoglobin SS) throughout the world will vary depending on the numbers of at-risk population and their particular gene frequency. The World Health Organization notes that the actual incidence of affected births varies greatly from one area to another. Their work, for example, suggests that the accepted 20–25 per cent incidence of heterozygotes for Hb S (carrier state) in parts of tropical Africa means that, in many areas, about 4 per cent of marriages are at risk of producing an affected child. They conclude that the high birth rate means that probably about 100,000 infants with sickle cell disease are born annually in the whole continent. This compares with about 1500 per year in the USA, 1600 per year in the Caribbean, 140 per year in the United Kingdom, and probably 4000 per year in South America (World Health Organization 1983: 65).

SC disease (haemoglobin SC)
A child born with SC disease has inherited a gene for sickle haemoglobin (Hb S) from one parent and a gene for haemoglobin C (Hb C) from the other parent. In his review of the distribution of sickle cell disorders Serjeant (1992) notes that the distribution of Hb C is much more limited, being primarily restricted to northern Ghana and Burkina Faso where the prevalence

of Hb C trait reaches as high as 20 per cent. With population movement, the frequency in the Caribbean and North America is found to be between 3.5 per cent and 2 per cent of the 'black' population respectively. The frequency of SC disease at birth can be as high as 1 in 50 in West Africa compared to 1 in 1000 in the North American black population and 1 per 500 births in Jamaica (Serjeant 1992).

Sickle beta thalassaemia
The two main types are sickle beta zero thalassaemia (SBeta^0), usually the more severe, and sickle beta plus thalassaemia (SBeta$^+$). From the available gene frequencies, Serjeant (1992) has calculated the crude incidence of both as approximately 1 in 800 in Ghana and 1 in 5000 births in the black population of North America. From his own Jamaican cohort study, the frequency of sickle beta plus thalassaemia was 1 in 3000 births and 1 in 7000 for sickle beta zero thalassaemia.

Signs, symptoms and management of sickle cell disorders

The underlying reason for many of the problems associated with sickle cell disorders centres on the capacity of the red blood cells to sickle under certain circumstances. This has become known as 'sickling' and applies to all the variations outlined above. Red cells sticking to the vessel lining is considered to be an important early step in vessel blocking due to excessive stickiness of the sickle haemoglobin-containing red blood cell. While there is still considerable debate on the underlying mechanisms (see for example Serjeant 1997) the sickling process is thought to distort the shape of the red blood cell into a half-moon or banana shape, causing two major complications:

1 sludging of the deformed red blood cells in the capillaries producing knots of red cells and thereby blocking the blood flow and causing tissue infarction. This results in a lack of oxygen to the tissues causing pain and damage to various organs in the body.
2 a faster destruction of red blood cells (haemolysis) due to the removal of the deformed sickled cells. The resulting chronic anaemia is due to this rapid breakdown of red blood cells and not to iron deficiency as commonly thought.

Table 3.1 outlines many of the factors that can trigger the sickling of the red blood cells. One or more of these factors can occur with anaesthetics, strenuous exercise, pregnancy and sudden cooling of the body that may occur when swimming in a poorly heated pool. Finally it is recognized that other, as yet unknown, causes as well as emotional factors may also be involved.

The clinical manifestations of sickle cell disorders are complex, variable in their severity and unpredictable in their presentation. Those with the condition are surviving longer but the quality of life is not always very good. While there have been some advances in treatment together with

Table 3.1   Factors that can cause sickling of the red blood cells

- Reduced amount of oxygen
- Lack of fluid (dehydration)
- Infection
- Sudden changes of temperature
- Acidosis
- Alcohol
- Smoking
- Stress

further developments on the horizon, the medical treatment of sickle cell disorders still presents a major challenge to health practitioners. Chapters 5 and 6 set out impact of this for affected individuals and their families. Here we focus on the general difficulties associated with the illness. The problems associated with sickle cell disorders – as we have seen – are generally unpredictable as well as variable in frequency and severity. This means that the complications we list are only probable and indeed some are extremely rare. Among the more common problems are pain, infections and anaemia. Other complications may include damage to various parts of the body depending upon where the sickling process takes place. Particular problem areas are the spleen, brain (e.g. strokes in early childhood), lungs, joints, particularly the hips and shoulders, penis (due to priapism, see later), spine, kidneys, ankles (leg ulcers) and eyes. Other problems include gallstones, haematuria (blood in the urine), jaundice, enuresis (bedwetting) and painful swelling of hands and feet in children (dactylitis or hand–foot syndrome). Common causes of death in early childhood include infections and severe anaemia, mainly due to problems in the spleen (such as splenic sequestration – a pooling of sickled blood). Chest syndrome (sickling in the lungs) accounts for the majority of deaths in young people and adulthood.

There are now many detailed reviews on sickle cell disorders which cover the variety of problems that can occur together with their management (Serjeant 1992; Department of Health 1993; Embury *et al.* 1994; Castro 1999; Davies and Oni 1997; Serjeant 1997; Steinberg 1999). In view of the numerous complications that are associated with SCD the following discussion will concentrate on just some of those that can result in frequent illness, disability and/or death.

Pain
A recurring theme occurring in the accounts of those affected by sickle cell disorders is the distress and suffering caused by the painful crisis and the impact this has on their relationships with family members and health workers (Anionwu and Beattie 1981; Black and Laws 1986; Murray and May 1988; Alleyne and Thomas 1994; National Health Service Management Executive 1994; Atkin *et al.* 1998a, 1998b; Maxwell *et al.* 1999). These

episodes of mild to excruciating episodes of pain are one of the commonest and most miserable aspects of the illness, affecting more than 70 per cent of those with SCD (Steinberg 1999). Minor pain crises are frequent and may be managed at home, with a high fluid intake, painkillers and soothing techniques such as gentle rubs with oils. Antibiotics are usually given if there is a fever or other evidence of underlying or precipitating infection. A study in the United States identified that a significant amount of pain was managed at home. Eighteen children and adolescents completed 4756 diary days with an average of 75 per cent compliance. Pain was reported on 30 per cent of days and nine out of ten times was managed at home, with girls reporting more pain than boys. There was an absence from school on 21 per cent of 3186 school days with half due to pain (Shapiro *et al.* 1995).

When the pain becomes unbearable, admission to hospital may be necessary for treatment with extremely strong analgesics such as morphine or pethidine. The painful crisis accounts for over 90 per cent of admissions for those with sickle cell disorders (Brozovic and Anionwu 1984; Brozovic *et al.* 1987). The pains can occur in any part of the body but frequently affect the limbs, back and chest. They may be local or generalized, fleeting or persistent. Some affected individuals sense the onset of a crisis (60 per cent in one study; Murray and May 1988), but it may also begin without any warning. The unpredictable onset and variable severity creates uncertainty and anxiety for the affected individual, their family and carers (see Chapter 5). Pain episodes can start in an infant as young as 3 to 6 months old but the highest rates of pain appear to occur between the ages of 19 and 39 years. However 40 per cent of patients in this same study had not had a painful crisis in any given year. This contrasted with 5 per cent of individuals who accounted for 30 per cent of all pain crises presenting to hospital (Platt *et al.* 1994). Individuals can have good and then bad patches. The pain may last a few hours or may persist for weeks with the average being a few days (Shapiro and Ballas 1994).

There is a body of literature that provides a catalogue of the varied conflicts and tensions between health workers and affected individuals concerning the management of the painful crisis (Baughan 1983; Murray and May 1988; Ballas 1990; Department of Health 1993; Shankleman and May 1993; Alleyne and Thomas 1994; National Health Service Management Executive 1994; Waldrop and Mandry 1995; Maxwell *et al.* 1999). They often find their pain inadequately treated due to various myths, stereotypes, low level of knowledge and lack of empathy. Pain management is an important site of struggle for people with SCD and this will be explored further in Chapters 5 and 6. Nonetheless, it might be useful to give some introduction to these difficulties. Ballas (1990) provides one of the most insightful accounts of pain management culled from his experience as a medical sickle cell specialist for over 15 years in Philadelphia. He focuses in particular on the small minority of patients (6–7 per cent) who accounted for a large percentage of emergency sickle cell care. A vivid picture is painted of the frustrations of patients because of long delays in the emergency room and then being seen by junior and inexperienced doctors. This is then made worse by accusations of being a 'junkie' and administration of inadequate doses of pain relief. He also details the fears of the doctors concerning the addictive nature of the powerful narcotics being demanded by the patients. Additionally they do not understand the use of distracting behaviour by patients (such as watching television, chatting with friends) while still complaining of pain. The patients' behaviour is cited as 'drug-seeking' whereas the patient would view it as 'pain-avoidance'.

This has been further corroborated in a study of health professionals concerning their perceptions of drug dependence of all patients (including those with sickle cell disorders) presenting to hospital (Waldrop and Mandry 1995). All of them estimated a higher percentage of drug dependency in sickle cell patients and far in excess of that shown in previous studies. The authors concluded that it was unknown whether pain medication was consequently withheld inappropriately by physicians. In terms of the British hospital experience, Maxwell *et al.* (1999) have provided an insight into the strategies developed by patients frequently admitted to hospital. They included the development of relationships with key staff, aggression, passivity and use of multiple hospitals. Chapters 5 and 6 will explore these issues in more detail.

In spite of the fact that the painful crisis accounts for so much illness and hospital admissions for those with sickle cell conditions, the present drug management is not based on any sound evidence. The Standing Medical Advisory Committee report noted that there had been 'no randomised clinical trials of opioid analgesic use in sickle cell crisis reported in the scientific literature' (Department of Health 1993: 43). One of the biggest problems has been deciding upon which is the best drug to treat the very severe episodes of pain. Davies (1991) recommended that it was time for coordinated trials of new treatments. Historically pethidine has been the drug of choice but reports of severe and sometimes fatal side effects (such as fits) with larger doses has led some units to switch to morphine or diamorphine (Ward *et al.* 1996). A very honest account has been provided by a north London haematologist about how this policy failed due to inadequate communication between patients and junior doctors (Yardumian 1993). The policy of utilizing a protocol and a multidisciplinary approach that included a systematic assessment and counselling of patients during each contact resulted in a 58 per cent decrease in emergency visits and a 44 per cent decrease in pain-related hospital admissions (Vichinsky *et al.* 1982). Guidelines on the management of both acute and chronic pain in sickle cell disorders have been produced in the United States (Benjamin *et al.* 1999) and these provide helpful guidance in a confused debate.

Infections
Infections represent the most common cause of deaths among infants and children with sickle cell disorders (Barrett-Connor 1971; Wong *et al.* 1992). The main reason is that the spleen, one of the key organs for fighting

infection, virtually stops functioning by early childhood. This can sometimes be reversed as a result of blood transfusions or bone marrow transplant. The infections are numerous and affect the chest (pneumonia), fluid surrounding the brain and spine (meningitis), bones (osteomyelitis) and the blood (septicaemia) with one of the main culprits being the pneumococcal bacteria. Over 80 per cent of pneumococcal infections occur between 6 months and 3 years of age and they are one of the commonest causes of death in young children with sickle cell anaemia (Rogers *et al.* 1978). The fact that the child had sickle cell anaemia was sometimes only diagnosed following post-mortem as the fatal infection was often the first major manifestation of the illness. This was ultimately recognized in the United States (Powars 1975), Jamaica (Rogers *et al.* 1978) and the UK (Ferriman 1984) and created the impetus to screen newborn babies before the onset of life-threatening problems.

There is now overwhelming evidence and consensus that neonatal screening, prophylactic penicillin from the age of 3 months, and parental education about the condition has significantly reduced deaths in this vulnerable age group (Powars *et al.* 1981; *Lancet* 1983; Gaston *et al.* 1986; Vichinsky *et al.* 1988; *Paediatrics* 1989; Sickle Cell Disease Guideline Panel 1993; Lee *et al.* 1995). When the affected children get older (usually after the age of 2 years) a pneumococcal vaccine may be administered to give added protection. Research is currently in progress to enable the vaccine in conjugated form to be given earlier than is possible at the moment. Evidence suggests that it is safe to stop penicillin prophylaxis at 5 years of age for children with sickle cell anaemia who have not had a prior severe pneumococcal infection or had their spleen removed. However they caution that parents must be aggressively counselled to seek medical attention whenever the affected child has a fever (Falletta *et al.* 1995).

The debate in Britain still centres on whether all babies should be screened or whether it should be targeted at certain ethnic groups. The Standing Medical Advisory Committee (Department of Health 1993) recommended universal neonatal screening in those districts where the antenatal population at risk of sickle cell disorders exceeded 15 per cent. This contrasts with the advice from an expert committee in the United States, which has advocated universal screening throughout the country. The committee suggested that, although the disorders are more prevalent in certain ethnic groups, it is not possible to define accurately an individual's origins by physical appearance or surname. They specifically pointed out the dangers of missing affected infants by targeting specific ethnic groups. To make neonatal screening programmes more cost-effective, the North American experience suggested that samples from low prevalence districts be analysed in laboratories in high prevalence ones rather than setting up their own service (Sickle Cell Disease Guideline Panel 1993). This has been reiterated in the two UK Health and Technology Assessment reviews on screening for sickle cell disorders (Zeuner *et al.* 1999; Davies *et al.* 2000). Chapter 4 explores the issue of screening in more detail.

Chest syndrome
This life-threatening complication arises due to sickling in the lungs, possibly combined with infection (Haynes *et al.* 1994; Vichinsky *et al.* 1997; Quinn and Buchanan 1999). It is a frequent cause of hospital admissions, second only to the painful crisis, and the commonest cause of death in older patients (Thomas *et al.* 1982). It affects between 15 and 43 per cent of individuals with sickle cell disorders, and 20 to 80 per cent will have repeated attacks. The symptoms include fever, coughing, chest pain, shortness of breath and worsening anaemia with audible crackles and/or bronchial breathing on examination of the chest, and often florid changes on chest X-ray. The patient may need assisted or mechanical ventilation. While there are thought to be many causes, the underlying features are not totally understood and treatment is often inadequate, although early detection and treatment may reduce severity and prevent death (Quinn and Buchanan 1999). Dramatic improvements have been noted following exchange blood transfusions.

Priapism
Sickling in the blood vessels of the penis, known as priapism, causes mild to excruciating painful erections and can result in impotence (Hakim *et al.* 1994). The age of onset can be as early as 5 years with peaks occurring from this age until 13 years of age and then from 21 to 29 years. Figures concerning frequency vary considerably from 10 to 40 per cent (Serjeant 1997; Steinberg 1999) to 64 per cent of 155 boys with SCD (Tarry *et al.* 1987). The variability in estimates is probably due in some part to embarrassment about the condition that may make it difficult for young males to discuss it with their parents and health care practitioners and a lack of awareness that it is in fact a complication of SCD. Mantadakis *et al.* (1999) undertook a survey among 98 male patients or their parents in a centre where 11 per cent were known to have experienced priapism, and discovered a further 18 per cent who had had one or more episodes. Treatment has ranged from increased fluids, relief of pain, surgery, drugs such as stilboestrol, transfusions and more recently, hydroxyurea. Impotence may be treated by a penile prosthetic implant (Serjeant 1997).

Complications that may result in a physical, visual or hearing impairment
As will be described in Chapters 5 and 6, many social services departments do not have SCD as one of their priorities in respect to chronic illness and disability. They are not aware of how the various problems associated with sickle cell disorders can result in a physical impairment for the affected child or adult.

Strokes are a particularly devastating complication that can occur in about 10 per cent of young children with sickle anaemia (Steinberg 1999). In Jamaica it had occurred in 7.8 per cent of children by the age of 14 years (Balkaran *et al.* 1992). The child may complain of weakness down one side and difficulty in speaking and walking. Prompt recognition of the problem is required to prevent further brain damage and physical impairment.

Recurrence of strokes is common, with rates being cited as between 46–90 per cent (R.J. Adams 1994). Treatment consists of immediate exchange blood transfusion to minimize extent of cerebral damage, then regular transfusions every four weeks to maintain Hb A level above 80 per cent. The duration of this form of treatment used to be about three years but this has lengthened and become open-ended because of high incidence of further strokes once blood transfusions are stopped.

Repeated blood transfusions, however, create an excess of iron in parts of the body such as the heart and the liver and this can lead to life-threatening complications. To prevent this problem a special drug that helps the body get rid of this excess iron has to be given by infusion (although research on an oral agent is underway). One such drug is desferrioxamine which, because it cannot be taken by mouth, has to be given by injection over a period of eight to twelve hours, five to seven nights a week. This is achieved through a battery operated syringe driver mechanism. The treatment is stressful and may be difficult for parents and affected individuals to comply with every day. (Although desferrioxamine treatment is a routine part of thalassaemia management, it is only necessary in the treatment of sickle cell disorders for those who have regular blood transfusions. A more detailed review of the complications associated with blood transfusions and the use of desferrioxamine appears in our discussion on thalassaemia.)

There is now some evidence for the utility of blood transfusions in preventing further strokes in those with sickle cell anaemia. Adams *et al.* (1998) enrolled 130 children with sickle cell anaemia who were identified to be at higher risk of stroke (through transcranial Doppler ultrasonography) into a multicentre study where 63 were randomly assigned to receive transfusions and 67 to receive standard care. As 11 children in the latter group had strokes compared to just one in the group being transfused, the study was terminated early. The authors concluded that prophylactic transfusions greatly reduced the risk of a first stroke but also acknowledged the long-term implications of iron overload and difficulties in coping with the treatment. Cohen (1998), in an accompanying editorial, reiterated these concerns and also pointed out that since nearly 40 per cent of the patients would be free of strokes without transfusions, they might have received transfusions needlessly for 10 years. Finally, Ware *et al.* (1999) have proposed that preliminary findings suggest that hydroxyurea may prevent recurrent strokes in some children and may be a better option than regular transfusions.

Further impairment can occur as a consequence of 'sickling' in the hips and shoulders. This is known as aseptic or avascular necrosis which results in degeneration of tissue within the joints and secondary arthritis, causing considerable pain and severe mobility problems for between 10 and 50 per cent of young adults with sickle cell anaemia and haemoglobin SC disease (Steinberg 1999). Total hip (and to a lesser extent, shoulder) replacement is a surgical intervention that may be offered where there is severe damage, but the operation may have to be repeated within a few years (Milner *et al.* 1994), particularly in young people, who are still developing.

Leg ulcers occur in up to 20 per cent of adults with sickle cell anaemia and management is still far from ideal, resulting in considerable pain, mobility problems, stigma, depression and disruption of education and employment (Cackovic *et al.* 1998; Steinberg 1999). A study in Jamaica (Alleyne *et al.* 1977) explored the social consequences of leg ulcerations in view of its high incidence among those with SCD. Three-quarters of individuals with sickle cell disorders in Jamaica are likely to develop leg ulceration during adolescence or in early adult life. Many UK experts consider that leg ulcers are rare in comparison with Jamaica but it must be noted that there appears to have been very little research undertaken here into the extent and impact of this complication. One exception is the work of Brozovic and Anionwu (1984) who noted that leg ulcers occurred in three people in Brent (4 per cent) in contrast with 40 in Jamaica (45 per cent). Castro (1999) notes that ankle ulcers in sickle cell disorders are probably related to chronic haemolysis (rapid destruction of red blood cells) rather than 'sickling' since similar ones occur in non-sickling haemolytic conditions such as thalassaemia intermedia and hereditary spherocytosis. He proposes that as hydroxyurea reduces the level of sickling in SCD it would appear reasonable to treat those with non-healing sickle ulcers with hydroxyurea as it reduces the level of haemolysis.

A variety of manifestations can arise also due to kidney problems. These include the inability to concentrate urine, leading to a higher rate of bedwetting (enuresis) in the young people; mild to severe episodes of blood in the urine (haematuria) often due to damage to the renal papillae known as renal papillary necrosis. This may lead to life threatening renal failure requiring kidney dialysis or transplantation. Renal failure occurs in 2.4 per cent of those with haemoglobin SC disease compared to 4.2 per cent of those with sickle cell anaemia (Powars *et al.* 1991) and patients also develop severe anaemia and high blood pressure.

Visual impairment can occur among those with SCD. Partial or total visual impairment can result from retinal sickling (proliferative sickle retinopathy) which is found in up to 33 per cent of individuals with haemoglobin SC disease and about 14 per cent of those with sickle cell anaemia (Castro 1999). Laser photocoagulation appears to be the preferred treatment but Castro comments that because of the relatively small number of patients enrolled in two randomized trials they were not in a position to answer all the efficacy and safety issues.

Hearing loss in SCD is thought to be due, among other reasons, to compression of the auditory nerve due to expansion of the bone marrow as well as possible damage to the cochlea due to the low oxygen tension that facilitates 'sickling' (Serjeant 1992). Studies among patients with SCD in various parts of the world have shown hearing loss to occur in 12 per cent of children in the USA, 21 per cent of children in Nigeria and 22 per cent of adults in Jamaica. This compares with control figures of 0.5 per cent, 7 per cent and 4 per cent respectively (Serjeant 1992). Health and social care staff are probably not adequately aware that hearing loss can be associated with SCD.

Pregnancy and contraception

As affected individuals now live longer, then more have entered into the reproductive age group. Historically there were reports of maternal death rates ranging between 20 and 50 per cent (Koshy and Burd 1994). Sterilization used to be recommended in the United States into the early 1970s because it was considered that sickle cell anaemia complicated pregnancy with a very poor prognosis for the mother and child (Fouche and Switzer 1949; Fort *et al.* 1971). Nearly 30 years later a prospective study in 19 US centres on the outcome of 445 pregnancies reported two deaths of mothers, one of which was directly related to her sickle cell disorder. The rate of sickle-related illness was the same as in the non-pregnant state. Twenty-one per cent of infants born to women with sickle cell anaemia were smaller than expected. The authors recommended that those caring for women with sickle cell disorders should support them if they want to have children (Smith *et al.* 1996). No similar prospective study has been undertaken in the United Kingdom – a paper in 1995 states that the maternal death rate is between 1 and 2 per cent (Howard and Tuck 1995). The impact on babies born to mothers with sickle cell disorders has been discussed in a paper by Howard *et al.* (1995). In a UK multicentre study a retrospective review of the outcome of such pregnancies noted a perinatal mortality rate of 60 per 1000 which compares to 8 per 1000 in the general obstetric population.

Until recently there has been conflicting advice on contraceptives for affected individuals. A study of 157 women with sickle cell disorders in North London (Howard *et al.* 1993) revealed the outcome of ad hoc and confusing advice concerning birth control. They found that only 29 per cent of their pregnancies were planned, 64 per cent were unplanned and 19 per cent were terminated for medical or social reasons, which indicated a serious lack of effective contraception and family planning advice. There is now much greater agreement that a variety of contraceptive techniques can be used, including the intrauterine device, injectable progesterones, such as Depo-Provera, the progesterone-only pill and even the combined oral contraceptive pills (Howard *et al.* 1993; Koshy 1995).

Recent advances in treatment

Bone marrow transplantation offer a potential 'cure' for SCDs (Vermylen *et al.* 1991) although – as we shall see – it is more commonly used in thalassaemia. The first successful bone marrow transplantation for sickle cell anaemia was performed in 1983 on an 8-year-old girl who also had leukaemia (Johnson *et al.* 1984). Ten years later almost 80 children had undergone the procedure with a rate of 5 per cent mortality and 90 per cent 'disease free survival' (Roberts 1994). It has to be remembered that the chance is 1 in 4 that any full brother or sister will be a suitable, tissue-type matched donor. In a report of bone marrow transplantation on 48 patients with sickle cell disorders, 42 (including four in whom the second transplant was successful) were reported to have disease-free survival (Mentzer 1994). Discussions have taken place concerning the ethics of offering bone marrow transplantation for sickle cell disorders in view of the risk of death or severe illness due to a rejection process called graft versus host disease (GVHD) (Smith 1992). Fertility is also impaired although pregnancies have been reported after bone marrow transplantation (Apperley 1993). Roberts (1994) suggests that it is reasonable to offer it to those children who fulfil the criteria set out in an international study of bone marrow transplantation for sickle cell disorders and this view is supported by Walters *et al.* (1996). A study of the attitudes of 67 parents of children with sickle cell disorders by Kodish *et al.* (1991) revealed that 54 per cent were willing to accept some risk of short-term mortality and 37 per cent the currently estimated 15 per cent mortality risk. Of considerable interest is the group of nine parents (13 per cent) who said they would accept a short-term mortality risk of 15 per cent or more and an additional 15 per cent risk of GVHD.

Bone marrow transplants using cord blood samples from a compatible newborn donor is emerging as a new development in this area (Kelly *et al.* 1997). This offers an exciting prospect that could greatly improve the treatment of SCD. Another possibility is gene therapy and this is discussed at the end of this chapter.

Hydroxyurea
A more recent development in management includes efforts to increase the level of fetal haemoglobin in order to reduce the severity of sickle cell disorders. A randomly controlled study with hydroxyurea was stopped before completion in view of the positive results (Charache *et al.* 1995). The researchers summarized the pros and cons of this treatment as follows:

> Hydroxyurea therapy can ameliorate the clinical course of sickle cell anaemia in some adults with three or more painful crises per year. The beneficial effects of hydroxyurea do not become manifest for several months, and its use must be carefully monitored. The long-term safety of hydroxyurea in patients with sickle cell anemia is uncertain.
> (Charache *et al.* 1995: 1317)

Sickle cell patients receiving hydroxyurea derived benefits that included a reduced number of episodes of pain and chest syndrome. They also required fewer blood transfusions and had an improved sense of well being, but hydroxyurea did not reduce the impact of strokes or death rates. Rodgers and Rachmilewitz (1995) reported an effective response rate in about 80 per cent of sickle cell patients receiving hydroxyurea. An initial multicentre study into safety aspects of administering hydroxyurea to children demonstrated sufficiently encouraging results to warrant the authors to advocate a trial to determine if hydroxyurea can prevent chronic organ damage (Kinney *et al.* 1999).

There are tensions, however, about the acceptability of hydroxyurea by those affected by SCD (see Consumers for Ethics in Research 1995) which centre on the concerns about long-term complications, inadequate explanation, feeling pressurized by doctors to take the drug and of being used as guinea pigs. The low uptake within the UK has been noted and debated in the medical journals (Davies and Roberts-Harwood 1998; Olujohungbe *et al*. 1998; Yardumian *et al*. 1999).

Survival

Due to improved survival sickle cell disorders can no longer be regarded as conditions that only affect children. While life expectation has greatly improved, the fear of death is still an understandable anxiety that is commonly experienced by affected families. It is best illustrated by the following comment from a nurse specialist in the United States: 'The fear of death is most prevalent. If the parents have heard anything at all about sickle cell, it is that their child will die . . . soon' (Jackson 1972: 738). This alarmist information can appear at the most unexpected times. A young adult with sickle cell anaemia attending the Brent centre, where Elizabeth Anionwu worked, recalled the fear experienced when, aged 16 years, she was taking the GCE Human Biology paper in 1973 (Associated Examining Board 1973). The first question concerned genetics and sickle cell anaemia was used as the example in the section on inheritance patterns. The description of the condition was 'Sickle-cells present, anaemia, death in childhood.' Chapter 5 discusses this in more detail.

Powars (1994b) states that 90 per cent of children with sickle cell anaemia born after 1980 and living in developing countries should reach the third decade of life. Evidence of increased life expectation comes from the cohort study in Jamaica (Lee *et al*. 1995) and the Co-operative Study of Sickle Cell Disease in the USA (Leikin *et al*. 1989; Platt *et al*. 1994). The Jamaican data is based on studying the progress of 315 children with sickle cell anaemia diagnosed at birth between June 1973 and December 1981. The groups were divided into three periods, the first born between June 1973 and December 1975 and the last third between January 1979 and December 1981. There were a total of 61 deaths before 15 years of age, 28 in the first group, 17 in the second and 16 in the last. Overall survival at 15 years was 73 per cent in the first group compared to 84 per cent in the third group. The reasons for this improvement included early diagnosis through neonatal screening and reduced deaths from acute splenic sequestration – probably due to parental education and removal of the spleen after two serious attacks, or after one if social circumstances were poor – and pneumococcal septicaemia and meningitis – following a trial of prophylactic penicillin.

Complications that still cause a significant number of deaths in this age group in Jamaica include infections due to haemophilus influenzae, the acute chest syndrome, aplastic crisis and strokes (Lee *et al*. 1995). Similar causes of death were noted in a prospective study in the USA of 703 children with sickle cell disorders born between October 1978 and October

1988 (Gill *et al.* 1995). Another American study found that approximately 85 per cent of children and young people with sickle cell anaemia and 95 per cent of patients with haemoglobin SC disease survived to 20 years of age (Leikin *et al.* 1989). In adults Platt *et al.* (1994) followed 3764 patients from birth to 66 years of age to determine life expectancy and calculate the median age at death. In addition they looked at the details of the 209 deaths that occurred during the study. The median age of death for children and adults with sickle cell anaemia was 42 years for males and 48 years for females. For those with haemoglobin SC disease it was 60 years for males and 68 years for females. They concluded that 50 per cent of patients with sickle cell anaemia survived beyond the fifth decade.

There have been no similar studies undertaken in the United Kingdom mainly because there is no comparable network of neonatal screening or any major cohort study as in Jamaica or the United States. A review of the scarce data available in the UK (Gray *et al.* 1991) ultimately concentrated on the Brent experience between 1974 and 1989 where there had been 18 deaths among a group of 384 patients. A worrying feature – noted in this review – concerned the number of centres reporting sudden deaths of people with sickle cell disorders. A special conference discussed the background to such deaths. The lack of any definitive causes prompted the recommendation that further research be undertaken (Liefner and Vandenberghe 1993).

Thalassaemia syndromes

In the final part of this chapter, we turn to thalassaemia. The first description of the clinical condition (but often called thalassaemia for shorthand as well as Cooley's or Mediterranean anaemia) is attributed to Dr Thomas Cooley and Dr Pearl Lee (Cooley and Lee 1925). They described their observations of children in the United States, primarily of Italian origin, who presented with anaemia, enlarged spleen and facial bone changes. There were many historical papers published during the 1930s, including the first recorded case in Britain in a Greek child (Moncrieff and Whitbey 1934). Whipple and Bradford (1936) described the illness as Mediterranean disease and also coined the term 'thalassaemia', from the Greek words for the sea and anaemia. Two years later Mukerji's paper (1938) was the first to describe the occurrence of the illness in those of Indian descent. The inheritance pattern was recognized by Caminopetros (1938) when he realized that both the parents and siblings of an affected child were carriers of a trait.

As previously described, the term thalassaemia indicates partial or no production of either the alpha or beta globin chains which form part of the structure of haemoglobin in the red blood cells (Weatherall 1997b). There are thus two main types: alpha thalassaemia and beta thalassaemia. This was first recognized by Ingram and Stretton (1959) and the different forms of alpha and beta thalassaemia are shown in Table 2.1.

The different types of thalassaemia

Alpha thalassaemia major
Alpha thalassaemia major, also known as hydrops fetalis, affects the unborn baby as it cannot make fetal haemoglobin which is made up of alpha and gamma globin chains. The latter requires four functioning genes which are located on two pairs. A fetus would normally inherit one pair from one parent and the remaining pair from the other. It is however possible for a person to be a carrier of alpha zero thalassaemia trait which means that they only possess two of these genes instead of four. While this does not affect their own health they can only pass on either their one pair of functioning genes or none at all. This becomes a problem when each parent is a carrier for alpha zero thalassaemia trait as their unborn baby can inherit alpha thalassaemia major when they both fail to pass on any alpha thalassaemia genes. This is incompatible with life and generally results in a miscarriage or stillbirth. The death of the fetus is due to an inability to produce haemoglobin and hence the development of the severe and fatal anaemia. The health of the mother is also in danger during the pregnancy as she may develop pre-eclampsia, a life-threatening increase in blood pressure that also causes fitting. Maternal deaths of this kind are avoidable if couples known to be from ethnic groups at risk of being carriers for alpha thalassaemia (such as those originating from Southeast Asia) are identified in early pregnancy (Petrou *et al.* 1992a, 1992b; Beris *et al.* 1995). It is then possible to offer testing on the unborn baby and/or arrange for ultrasound scanning to detect any changes in the normal development of the fetus. The risk is present in every subsequent pregnancy but, as couples are not always identified, recommendations for screening policies have been outlined (Petrou *et al.* 1992a, 1992b).

H disease
This moderately severe anaemia, but usually well compensated (Weatherall 1997b) occurs when a child inherits only one of the four alpha thalassaemia genes but, unlike alpha thalassaemia major, is not fatal to the unborn baby. The degree of anaemia does vary and affected individuals are prone to having an enlarged spleen, particularly at times of infections. As a result they need advice if taking part in sporting activities to ensure the spleen does not rupture following excessive physical contact. Occasionally removal of the spleen may be required but on the whole their quality of life and survival chances are not greatly impaired. In fact some are only diagnosed as adults following a routine blood test that reveals small red blood cells and the presence of 'H' bodies on a specially stained blood film.

Beta thalassaemia major
Beta thalassaemia major, unlike alpha thalassaemia major that affects the unborn baby, is a life threatening anaemia that generally starts after 3 months of age. There are numerous mutations giving rise to thalassaemia

beta genes, normally categorized as beta plus ($^+$) thalassaemia and beta zero (^{0}) thalassaemia. The two main forms of the condition are beta thalassaemia major and beta thalassaemia intermedia. Beta thalassaemia major is defined by the affected individual being dependent on regular blood transfusions for survival. This is because, in the absence of treatment, the condition will result in a fatal anaemia due to the partial or total absence of haemoglobin. Beta thalassaemia intermedia is described below.

Beta thalassaemia intermedia and E beta thalassaemia
While beta thalassaemia major is more common, there are also individuals with other types of thalassaemia, such as beta thalassaemia intermedia (Ratip *et al.* 1995; Ho *et al.* 1998) and E beta thalassaemia (Glader and Look 1996, Fucharoen and Winichagoon 2000). It has been estimated that the relative frequency of thalassaemia intermedia ranges from 2 to 10 per cent of thalassaemia cases in different populations. Thalassaemia intermedia is generally a milder condition than that usually associated with beta thalas- saemia major. The individual, for instance, does not usually require life- long regular blood transfusions in order to survive (Modell and Berdoukas 1984), although some people may require transfusion management. Further, the affected person may still experience bone changes, anaemia, leg ulcers and delayed development (Weatherall 1997b) as well as psycho- social consequences approaching those for beta thalassaemia major (Ratip *et al.* 1995). Factors that may result in beta thalassaemia intermedia include the inheritance of mild beta$^+$ thalassaemia mutations, the co-inheritance of alpha thalassaemia and the inheritance of factors that enhance the gamma- globin gene expression (Wainscoat *et al.* 1987). Beta thalassaemia intermedia is not always straightforward to diagnose but this is gradually improving due to the significant amount of knowledge now available about the genetic basis of this disorder (Ratip *et al.* 1995). However it is not always possible to predict the clinical severity from genetic analysis alone (Ho *et al.* 1998). E beta thalassaemia is also a milder form of the beta thalassaemia syn- drome and again, affected individuals are not usually dependent on monthly blood transfusions.

Signs, symptoms and management

A child with beta thalassaemia major appears to be perfectly well at birth. This is because, like all newborns, the majority of haemoglobin at this age is of the normal fetal kind. The problems start after 3 to 6 months of age when the body attempts the normal switchover to the production of adult haemoglobin. This is not possible in beta thalassaemia major and therefore the child starts to develop an anaemia that will become progressively worse (Weatherall and Clegg 1981; Modell and Berdoukas 1984).

Problems are usually apparent by the age of 2 years and often much younger, sometimes by 6 months of age (Vullo *et al.* 1995). In the absence of diagnosis and regular blood transfusions, typical signs and symptoms of the illness will include failure to thrive, pallor, poor appetite, vomiting, irritability and difficulty in sleeping. The child may also have a fever and an enlarged abdomen due to an increased spleen (Modell and Berdoukas 1984). The bone marrow of the child will work overtime in a desperate attempt to produce haemoglobin. As a result it expands and produces the prominent forehead known as 'bossing'. The majority of untransfused patients will die during their first two years of life, and often much younger, sometimes by 6 months of age, as the severe anaemia will cause complications such as heart failure, bossing, maxilliary expansion and dental problems (Piomelli 1995).

Treatment with regular blood transfusions has dramatically improved the survival of those born with beta thalassaemia major (Olivieri *et al.* 1994). However these transfusions also contain iron which cannot be excreted at all from the body. It therefore accumulates to dangerous levels in various organs such as the heart and liver. The introduction of drugs to get rid of this excess iron (chelating agents) has done much to reduce this life-threatening problem (also see above). The one licensed drug to remove iron from the body is desferrioxamine, which is inactive by mouth and has to be given parenterally. Nonetheless, the use of the slow infusion pump to inject this type of drug into the body is not straightforward. Early deaths, due to iron-overload, occur in a significant number of young adults who have found it extremely difficult to keep up with daily injections into their abdomen or thighs (Atkin and Ahmad 2000c; Modell *et al.* 2000b). In addition there may be side-effects of chelating drugs such as desferrioxamine (Desferal[R]) that are used to remove excess iron from the body. The oral chelator deferriprone is available on a named patient basis, but not licensed. There are some worrying side-effects, in particular, sudden falls in the neutrophil count (a type of white blood cell that helps to fight infections), need careful monitoring. Despite these problems, improved survival has demonstrated that beta thalassaemia major is no longer exclusively a childhood illness. One consequence of improved life expectation has been to reveal the complications that can affect an individual as they get older. A summary of the main problems that may occur in a person with a beta thalassaemia syndrome are outlined in Table 3.2.

Treatment and management

The essence of managing the condition, as we have seen, is regular blood transfusions for life (Piomelli 1995), preventing or treating the potentially fatal complication of iron-overload (Giardina and Grady 1995) and dealing with the various other manifestations of the illness. A more recent development for this condition is bone marrow transplantation (Lucarelli *et al.* 1995) which, when successful, can cure the condition (also see above). The Thalassaemia International Federation (TIF) has distributed two useful booklets on the management of the condition, one for affected individuals (Vullo *et al.* 1995) and the other for health professionals (Cappellini *et al.* 2000).

In order to combat life-threatening anaemia, a child with beta thalassaemia major will require regular blood transfusions for life. Early treatment

Table 3.2   Problems that may occur in a person with beta thalassaemia major

---

Transfusion related

Undertransfusion
• Severe, life threatening anaemia
• Bone marrow expansion
• Enlarged spleen

Transfusion
• infections (from a variety of sources particularly viral ones transmitted through blood transfusions. They include hepatitis B & C and HIV)
• organ damage from iron-overload or infection (leading to heart and liver failure)

Damage to endocrine glands
• Diabetes
• Hypothyroidism
• Hypoparathyroidism
• Delay in puberty and fertility problems

Other
• Bone complications such as osteoporosis which may result in collapse of the spine

---

was extremely conservative and blood transfusions were given irregularly. Piomelli (1995) notes that the first doctor to introduce a more regular regime was Orsini in Marseilles (Orsini and Boyer 1961). In 1964 Wolman, a paediatrician based in Philadelphia, described the findings of a survey of transfusion programmes in clinics on the eastern seaboard of the United States (Wolman 1964). There was a significant improvement in the quality of life of children who had been regularly transfused. In particular, the embarrassing facial features associated with bossing could be prevented if transfusions were started early in life. The period between blood transfusions may range from two to four weeks but there is still debate about the ideal interval (Piomelli 1995). All UK blood is now filtered by the National Blood Authority because of the risk of New Variant CJD. Most children with beta thalassaemia major develop an enlarged spleen by the age of 8 or 9 years especially if they are undertransfused. This will increase the amount of blood required by the body. Others have a high blood consumption even when the spleen is not enlarged; in either case, removal of the spleen should be considered. When the volume reaches a certain level, removal of the spleen (splenectomy) is recommended. The spleen helps to fight infections and therefore after the operation it will be necessary for the person to be protected by vaccination and by taking penicillin for life. This, as we have seen, is also a common strategy among those with SCD.

Blood transfusion programmes should aim to cause the least disruption as possible to the normal everyday routine of the child or adult. This ideally requires day units with designated beds, which are open during the evening and at weekends to enable continued attendance at school, college or work.

The staff of the unit should include trained clinical nurse specialists who can speedily put up the blood transfusion. This avoids patients having to wait hours for a doctor who is elsewhere attending to emergencies and other more 'acute' situations. Chapter 6 explores these issues in greater detail.

Various problems are associated with blood transfusions and these include – as we have seen – iron overload and viral infections. We begin by discussing iron overload, the more common of the problems. A patient with beta thalassaemia major may be transfused with 25–30 units of blood a year and with each unit they also receive approximately 180 mg of iron (Piomelli 1995). It has been estimated that a 12-year-old patient receiving appropriate transfusions will have stored 55 or more grams of excess iron in various tissues that would normally have approximately 2 grams (Giardina and Grady 1995). An additional cause of iron overload is that iron is absorbed from the gastrointestinal tract at a faster than normal rate. Iron damage to the heart is the commonest cause of death. Other complications include damage to the liver, increased pigmentation of the skin and endocrine problems (Jensen and Tuck 1994).

These endocrine problems include pancreatic damage, resulting initially in impaired glucose tolerance. This does not require insulin but attention to diet, weight and exercise. It may develop into insulin dependent diabetes (which occurs in approximately 6 to 8 per cent of patients). Treatment with insulin adds yet another burden for those already needing to inject themselves to use the pump as self-infusion with desferrioxamine is commonly called. Two other common problems associated with the endocrine system are short stature due to immature growth and impaired sexual development resulting in infertility. Historically it was assumed that women with beta thalassaemia major would never be able to have children. There are now reports of several who have had successful pregnancies, many following ovulation treatment (Jensen *et al.* 1995). Other endocrine conditions include hypothyroidism and hypoparathyroidism. Finally, another important problem concerns bone complications such as osteoporosis that may cause spontaneous fractures.

Prevention and management of iron overload became possible with the advent, over 20 years ago, of the chelating agent, desferrioxamine. One major drawback was that it was not effective when taken by mouth and the initial suggestion of intravenous use was not considered practical (Giardina and Grady 1995). In the mid-1970s research demonstrated that intramuscular injections of desferrioxamine, six days a week, enabled significant excretion of iron in the urine (Letsky 1976). An important milestone occurred a few years later with the development of a small battery-driven infusion pump through which the drug could be given sub-cutaneously (Propper *et al.* 1977). This is now the commonest method used to prevent transfusion-acquired iron overload. Young children are taught from an early age to put a small needle under the skin in the abdomen or thigh. This is connected to a piece of fine tubing that is attached to a syringe filled with a solution of desferrioxamine powder previously mixed with distilled water. The syringe is placed in the battery operated pump that controls the rate at

Table 3.3   Possible side-effects of desferrioxamine

- Irritation at the site of injecting the drug. This can cause mild to severe inflammation as well as the development of hard lumps under the surface. More recently it has been recognized that patients using certain batches of the drug were experiencing much more severe local reactions. As a result the manufacturer, Ciba-Geigy, altered some aspects of their production method.
- Generalized reactions are less commonly reported than localized ones. They appear to be due to an allergic-type response and include symptoms of dizziness, breathing difficulties and a general sense of being unwell. They tend to start when a person first starts the drug and can often be overcome by a desensitization programme. However a few people will not be able to tolerate the drug and have to be switched to another chelating agent. This can also be given through the pump but in addition the person also needs to take a zinc supplement. They need to have regular checks to ensure that they are not suffering from any complications due to a lack of this mineral.
- Too high a dose can cause a variety of problems including high tone deafness and visual impairment. If these problems occur it is usual to stop the drug and consider using an oral chelator instead.
- Certain infections that are not usually severe can become very serious, and even fatal, in those taking desferrioxamine. An important example is yersinia enterocolitica, an infection that can result in fever, diarrhoea and abdominal pain. Anyone experiencing these symptoms is advised to immediately stop taking desferrioxamine and seek medical attention as soon as possible (Vullo *et al*. 1995).

---

which the drug is then infused into the body over eight to twelve hours, five to seven nights a week. For those who find the injections too painful, a local anaesthetic preparation (such as Emla cream) can be applied on to the skin about an hour before inserting the needle. Inability to tolerate such a regimen, as we shall see, is still a major problem. It has been noted that vitamin C, given in addition to desferrioxamine, can increase the amount of iron excreted from the body. The use of desferrioxamine resulted in a striking improvement in the survival of those born with thalassaemia major after 1960 (Modell *et al*. 1982; Zurlo *et al*. 1989). There are, however, a variety of recognized side-effects of desferrioxamine, which are set out in Table 3.3.

Despite the obvious advantages of the pump it is understandable why a significant number of individuals – particularly young people – have difficulty in keeping up with the demanding treatment (this will be explored further in Chapter 5). As a result they succumb to the effects of iron overload in the form of heart or liver failure. These complications are now one of the main causes of death in beta thalassaemia major (Davies and Wonke 1991; Apperley 1993; Modell *et al*. 2000b). Giardina and Grady (1995: 310) make a plea that 'significant attention should be paid to new strategies aimed at fostering improved compliance with its use'. Historically, serum ferritin levels have been measured to provide some idea about the extent of iron-overload. Liver iron concentration (ascertained by methods such as liver biopsy or an MRI) is now being advocated as a more reliable alternative to serum ferritin (Capellini *et al.* 2000).

The UK Thalassaemia Society has recognized the difficulties experienced with the pump and the need to develop a tablet that can be taken by mouth. As a result they raised sufficient funds to initiate trials with oral drugs such as deferiprone, also known as L1. The first clinical trials started in 1987 and extended to other parts of the world such as India (Mavroudis 1990). Although adequate amounts of iron appear to be removed there are reports of toxicity, particularly a severe reduction in white blood cells, known as agranulocytosis. This has required further studies prior to the possibility of wider use (Olivieri 1996) but conflicts then arose between the Canadian pharmaceutical company and the key researcher Dr Nancy Olivieri concerning the findings and their dissemination. The episode has been cited as an example of problems that can occur when there may be conflicts of interest between academics and the commercial sector (see for example Nathan and Weatherall 1999). This is part of the wider context in which strategy and struggle occur.

In the meantime options, when compliance is poor, include delivery of desferrioxamine directly into the circulation through a permanent insertion of a Hickman or a Port-a-Cath line intravenously or into a central vein. This is usually in the chest area, and great care is required to avoid the major risk of infections following the introduction of such catheters. However, this can reverse or improve even quite severe heart dysfunction and can be life saving.

Viral infections
We now turn to a second complication associated with thalassaemia: viral infections. The ability of the human immunodeficiency virus to be acquired from blood transfusions has helped to publicize other blood-borne viruses such as hepatitis B and particularly hepatitis C. Individuals with conditions requiring regular treatment with blood products, such as those with haemophilia or beta thalassaemia major, are particularly vulnerable. The introduction of screening of blood and other measures has now significantly reduced the risk of transmitting certain viruses. However those receiving blood prior to the introduction of these measures have been at considerable risk. A review in the mid-1990s has shed light on the numbers of those affected, particularly in Europe (de Montalembert *et al.* 1995).

In the mid to late 1980s the figures ranged from 2 to 11 per cent of patients infected with HIV in Italy and Greece compared to 12 per cent in the United States. They were mainly infected before the introduction of systematic screening of blood donations. A more recent investigation followed a group of 2972 patients in 14 European and Mediterranean countries who had no evidence of HIV infection at the beginning of the study in January 1988. A year later, further tests did not find any indication of infection in this period as there was no evidence of HIV seroconversion (Lefrere *et al.* 1989). A similar study following 1305 patients in Italy between

December 1989 and November 1990 found a residual risk of HIV infection to be 1 in 50,000 blood units (Mozzi *et al.* 1992).

Liver failure is the second commonest cause of death and is due to hepatitis B and C transmitted through blood transfusions (Davies and Wonke 1991). While jaundice may occur, most people do not suffer a major acute illness when they first become infected with hepatitis B. Blood donors should be routinely screened for this virus and individuals with beta thalassaemia major need to receive the hepatitis B vaccine before they ever start having blood. Despite the possibility of these preventive measures, post-transfusion infection still occurs. A significant number of patients negative for the virus have still not received the vaccine (de Montalembert *et al.* 1995).

Hepatitis C virus was only identified in 1989 and it has been estimated that about 25 per cent of patients in the United Kingdom and 40 per cent in the Mediterranean have been infected by hepatitis C virus via blood transfusions (Cao *et al.* 1992). One of the highest figures noted in a review of viral complications (de Montalembert *et al.* 1995) came from a 1992 study in Italy which found the virus in 72 per cent of thalassaemic patients (Rebulla *et al.* 1992). Approximately half will go on to be affected by chronic hepatitis (inflammation of the liver). A further 20 per cent of this group will develop cirrhosis of the liver and of these a further 20 per cent are at risk of developing life-threatening liver tumours. About half of those with hepatitis C will respond to the drug interferon, but half of this group will relapse once they stop the treatment (Donahue *et al.* 1993). A more encouraging response has been observed in this latter group of patients who are subsequently treated with a combination of interferon-alpha and ribavirin. One side-effect is that their blood transfusion requirements are increased (Wonke *et al.* 1996).

Bone marrow transplantation

While there have been significant advances in the management of beta thalassaemia it is still a chronic illness that can cause early death or a diminished quality of life. As a result, consideration was given to more dramatic and riskier interventions such as bone marrow transplants. Bone marrow transplantation is more commonly undertaken for beta thalassaemia major than sickle cell anaemia as the latter has a less predictable clinical outcome. The first successful bone marrow transplant on someone with thalassaemia was undertaken in 1982 on a 14-month-old untransfused child (Thomas *et al.* 1982). Weatherall (1993) recalls the lack of enthusiasm for bone marrow transplants as a means of curing the condition, mainly due to the initial poor outcome of the technique. His suggestion that the more encouraging results, particularly from the Pesaro group in Italy, make this therapy a genuine option for the management of severe forms of beta thalassaemia have now been realized (Lucarelli *et al.* 1998).

Lucarelli, a leading pioneer from Pesaro, began to obtain outstanding successes by observing which patients were more likely to survive. As a result he divided patients into three prognostic categories according to risk factors (the best being class one, the worst class three), the most important being the size of the liver and regular use of iron chelation. Between June 1983 and December 1994 the group had undertaken 697 transplants (Lucarelli *et al.* 1995), 111 in class one, 294 in class two and 165 in class three. The overall 'cure' rate was 72 per cent and 20 per cent died. The results according to class categories were respectively: cured – 100 (one), 239 (two) and 93 (three). Deaths from causes related to the transplant were: 4 (one), 42 (two) and 46 (three).

As discussed earlier in relation to sickle cell disorders, an encouraging development has been the ability to transplant an individual using the compatible cord blood from a newborn baby (Hutchinson 1994; Thompson 1995). The advantages include a lower risk of rejection and a possible faster way of finding a donor because of the establishment of cord blood banks.

In the UK, according to Professor Bernadette Modell (personal communication), by the second half of 1998 there had been 110 bone marrow transplants, with 87 disease-free survivors (representing 25 per cent of patients born since 1985). There were four recurrences of thalassaemia and three cases of chronic graft–versus–host disease. Sixteen of the 22 deaths among patients born since 1980 were associated with bone marrow transplantation. There are continued concerns voiced in Britain about the impression that might be given to parents that this is the obvious therapy for their child with a beta thalassaemia disorder. Initial results at some British centres were not as good as those in Italy (Vellodi *et al.* 1994) and this may be one of the reasons for the concerns that still exist among some professionals in Britain. They centre on the risks of transplant related mortality in this condition, for which – unlike the malignant conditions for which transplant is more often undertaken – there is available continued conventional therapy.

Finally bone marrow transplantation does not alter the genetic make-up of the individual. As a result genetic counselling is required to ensure that the person understands that they will always pass on the gene for beta thalassaemia, if they remain fertile post-transplant. It is only if their partner is a carrier of beta thalassaemia that any of their children have a chance of inheriting the illness.

The management and treatment of beta thalassaemia intermedia
The variability of this condition was confirmed by a study of 28 patients and their parents undertaken in London to evaluate the psychosocial burden of thalassaemia intermedia (Ratip *et al.* 1995). The age at diagnosis varied from birth to 19 years plus one person who was not diagnosed until age 54 following complaints of lethargy. One-third (31 per cent) had not had any blood transfusions while the remaining 69 per cent were receiving regular transfusions every three to twelve months. Leg ulcers were experienced by 23 per cent and over half (58 per cent) of the patients had problems with sexual development. Half (51 per cent) had some degree of facial

deformity and 42 per cent had some degree of mobility problem. This ranged from weakness on walking that required periodic rests to being unable to walk more than half a mile or climb more than 10 stairs. The authors found that 81 per cent of the parents interviewed would have chosen prenatal diagnosis if it had been available and would have terminated all affected pregnancies.

Survival

In Italy the survival data on 1146 patients with beta thalassaemia major born between 1 January 1960 and 31 December 1987 was studied (Borgna-Pignatti *et al.* 1998). At the last follow-up in March 1997 the probability of survival to 20 years of age was 89 per cent and for those born between 1970 and 1974, 82 per cent survived to 25 years of age. The authors noted that patients who died had a significantly higher serum ferritin level one year before their death than those who survived.

In 1998 the UK Thalassaemia register comprised 820 patients with a diagnosis of beta thalassaemia major, including 24 who have been lost to follow-up, representing over 95 per cent of these people with thalassaemia major ever born or resident in the UK (Modell *et al.* 2000b). Of the remaining 796 patients, 190 (24 per cent) were known to be deceased. To study survival in more depth, and relate it to the historical developments in treatment, patients over the age of 12 years were divided into four 10-year birth cohorts (see Table 3.4).

The early deaths were mainly due to the original inadequate transfusion therapy and initial complications of bone marrow transplantation, but these have fallen from 30 per cent to 2.8 per cent. The majority of deaths of those over 12 years of age were as a result of heart failure due to transfusional iron overload with up to 50 per cent of patients appearing to have major problems in tolerating the use of the desferrioxamine infusion pump.

Gene therapy – a future therapy for sickle cell and thalassaemia disorders?

Prior to concluding this chapter on the complications and management of sickle cell and thalassaemia disorders, the possible role of gene therapy for

Table 3.4   The status of 748 UK patients with beta thalassaemia major (born between 1945–1994)

- 1945–1954: 21 (84 per cent) out of 25 of the most senior age group
- 1955–1964: 67 (56 per cent) out of 119 patients
- 1965–1974: 63 (34 per cent) out of 188 patients
- 1975–1984: 33 (14 per cent) out of 237 patients
- 1985–1994: 5 (3 per cent) out of 179 patients

both of these conditions will be explored. It is not surprising that sickle cell and thalassaemia disorders were among the first conditions to be considered as serious candidates for gene therapy (Sadelain 1997). However the initial hopes of the early 1980s have not yet been realized due to a variety of problems (Emery and Stamatoyannopoulos 1999). These include the capture and expansion of haemopoietic stem cells that are seen as the ideal cell for gene therapy for haemoglobinopathies. Other difficulties are associated with identifying the most effective method for both the transfer and expression of the gene. Developments continue and cautious optimism is being expressed in the scientific literature (see Blouin *et al.* 2000; Howrey *et al.* 2000) that gene therapy still offers the best possibility of effecting a cure for the haemoglobinopathies.

Conclusion

The aim of this chapter has been to provide a comprehensive overview of the clinical problems of sickle cell and thalassaemia disorders together with their management. This has included symptoms, life expectation, current treatment and future prospects. While there have been important developments in the management of the conditions one of the saddest ironies is that these significant scientific advances have not yet been translated into generally acceptable treatment regimens. For those with SCD this centres particularly on inadequate management of pain while for those with thalassaemia syndromes it is the difficulties surrounding the use of the desferrioxamine infusion pump. The subsequent chapters will build on this understanding and examine the social context of sickle cell and thalassaemia. Our analysis will begin by exploring genetic screening and counselling.

4

Genetic screening and counselling: ethics, politics and practice

For those at risk of a haemoglobinopathy, prenatal and antenatal screening as well as population screening to identify carriers is available, to varying degrees, in most parts of the UK (Anionwu 1993; Bain and Chapman 1998). The coverage, however, is extremely patchy (Modell and Anionwu 1996). As a consequence of ad hoc screening policies, children are often not identified until some time after birth (Davies *et al.* 1993) and evidence suggests that carrier detection and screening in pregnancy is uncoordinated (Department of Health 1993, Modell *et al.* 2000a). Further, counselling, either at the time of diagnosis or during carrier testing is rarely related to individual need (Atkin and Ahmad 1997). Screening and counselling provision therefore raises a variety of problems, the consequences of which range from the denial of informed choice to avoidable suffering, as well as risk of earlier death for some undiagnosed children (Darr 1990; Atkin *et al.* 1998b; Modell *et al.* 2000a). Many of these problems reflect the generally poor quality provision offered to carriers and those with the illness alike and whilst discussing them we will explore many of the themes in subsequent chapters.

This analysis, however, must be further grounded within the broader social and political context. Such a grounding ensures that debate about haemoglobinopathies does not become marginalized. As the opening chapter argued, discussions about sickle cell and thalassaemia implicate many general issues, such as the status of minority ethnic groups as citizens, racism and developing appropriate and successful provision to minority ethnic groups (Darr 1999; Dyson 1999). An explanation of issues around sickle cell and thalassaemia therefore allows us to explore other general concerns, such as demands, equity, access and the value of political engagement on the one hand, and notions of deservingness based on racialized constructions of citizenship on the other.

Another general theme of this chapter is the growing importance of the 'new genetics'. As inherited recessive disorders, haemoglobinopathies are implicated in the growing fascination about the genetic basis of disease and the development of provision to identify such conditions (Bradby 1996). Such provision necessarily covers a varied set of practices aimed at a varied set of people. The genetic element in disease, for example, ranges from single gene defects that can cause major disorders to genetic predispositions to genetic influences in conditions such as congenital malformation, cancer, diabetes, coronary heart disease and mental health problems (Modell *et al.* 1991; Harper 1998). Nonetheless, common issues emerge. For example, one of the most contested areas for most genetic screening and counselling programmes is the degree to which informed choice is truly available to those at risk of having a child with an inherited disorder (Chadwick 1993).[1] The emerging tension between 'informed decision-making' and 'disease prevention' is at the heart of the 'new genetics' and is where we begin our discussion.

Haemoglobinopathies and the 'new genetics'

NHS provision for identifying 'at risk' couples, affected unborn children and newborn babies is now available for haemoglobinopathies (Royal College of Physicians 1989). As with all provision for recessive disorders, these services emphasize the importance of providing information to enable at-risk couples to make an informed choice in reproductive decisions and to support and care for children born with the condition (Davies *et al.* 1993, 2000; see also Nuffield Council on Bioethics 1993 and Science and Technology Committee 1995 for a broader discussion of these issues). However, the influence of medical discourses on the 'new genetics' also introduces an idea, often implicit, of prevention (Atkin and Ahmad 1997). Thalassaemia, for example, is often described as a 'preventable condition', whose incidence can be reduced by implementing a programme of health education and genetic counselling (Pallister 1992). The tension between informed decision-making and prevention is thus fundamental in understanding the 'new genetics'. The comments of the late Cedric Carter, who played a significant role in the development of clinical genetic services in Britain, reflect this. In an article discussing the principle generally adopted in genetic counselling clinics he states: 'ultimate decisions on whether to take the risk of having a child with a genetic defect must rest with the husband and wife' (Carter 1979: 1794). He, however, concluded: 'The long-term aim of genetic counselling is to see that as few children as possible are born with serious genetically determined or part genetically determined handicaps' (1979: 1798).

The tension as to whether prevention is the objective of screening for genetic conditions is illustrated in the differing views in reports commissioned by the NHS Research and Development Health and Technology Assessment (HTA) programme in respect to population screening: 'The aim of genetic screening for cystic fibrosis is to reduce the birth prevalence of the disorder' (Murray *et al.* 1999); and 'the principle aim of screening for fragile-X syndrome is to reduce the birth prevalence of the disorder' (Murray *et al.* 1997). These views are in contrast with those who perceive the object-ive of screening to be that of facilitating informed decision-making (see Pembrey *et al.* 2001, in respect to fragile-X).

Debates on haemoglobinopathies specifically embody this problem. Policy documentation, for instance, rarely articulates the tension, emphasizing instead the importance of informed decision-making, and its impact on the reduction of affected births (Department of Health 1993; Health Education Authority 1998). Further, the dramatic fall in affected births in Cyprus has (wittingly or not) promoted the idea that a 'successful' haemoglobinopathy screening programme can be measured by the reduction in the number of affected births (see Ashiotis *et al.* 1973; Angastiniotis and Hadjimanas 1981; Kuliev 1986). This idea finds expression in UK policy and Petrou and Modell (1995: 1285), although emphasizing the importance of informed choice, conclude: 'Since the demand for prenatal diagnosis is very high in European and Mediterranean countries, a rough but good indicator of the delivery of services is the fall in the thalassaemia birth rate'.

Practice guidance further reflects this tension. Health commissioners, for example, similarly emphasize the importance of informed decision-making in the practice guidance and the general importance of empowerment (Atkin *et al.* 1998b). At the same time, genetic counselling services are often sold to health commissioners on the understanding that a significant proportion of prospective parents will make the 'right decision' and abort affected children. Indeed to help health service managers in this analysis, there are costing models demonstrating the cheaper costs of screening compared to the costs of providing life-long care for a child affected with a haemoglobin-opathy (Ostrowsky *et al.* 1985). These views of a health commissioner, commenting on the purpose of counselling, specially illustrate this tension: 'Empowering them [parents] to make their own decisions. And to *prevent* by giving people an *informed choice*' (cited in Atkin *et al.* 1998b: 1646; emphasis added).

To prevent by giving an informed choice

To understand fully the tension between *informed decision-making* and *prevention*, it is important to explore the various ideas that come to inform the origins and development of the 'new genetics'. Admittedly, any descrip-tion of these ideas is necessarily a caricature. Nonetheless, they have ana-lytical value in summarizing the main themes of the 'new genetics'. More generally, understanding these ideas is not simply an academic exercise but can inform the strategies and struggles of those committed to improving existing provision. To this extent, our discussion can be seen as a ground-clearing exercise, identifying opportunities for action as well as potential threats to emancipatory activity (see Bauman 1992).

Essentially the 'new genetics' becomes informed by two different themes that appear contradictory (Atkin and Ahmad 1997). On the one hand, a discourse looks to prevent disease in order to maximize human satisfaction and well-being. On the other, there is a discourse emphasizing the importance of the active human agency, exercising control over one's own life. In practice the two themes become interwoven and impossible to separate, part of the taken-for-granted background to providing genetic services. In turn, these themes cannot escape the influence of ideas about scientific medicine and public health, humanism, eugenics, consumerism and citizenship. All these ideas come to influence the debate about genetic and screening services available to those at risk of a haemoglobinopathy. The subsequent debate, however, is far from consistent and reflects various influences, offering solution as well as paradox as they celebrate the complexity of social life (see Bourdieu 1977).

In western industrial societies, 'scientific medicine' is the dominant paradigm within which to construct, interpret and deal with disease (Scambler 1987). The 'new genetics' grew directly from this tradition as scientific medicine looked to increase its knowledge of the biochemical process in explaining the aetiology of disease and then using this understanding to 'cure' affected individuals. Accordingly, the social role of the doctor is one of active expert sanctioned by the state on society's behalf, and the role of the patient has been one of a passive non-expert who must comply with medical investigations and treatment. Genetic status can thus be objectively gauged within the body.

The 'new genetics' is also grounded in another important aspect in the development of medical discourse: public health. As medicine recognized the social, economic and environmental determinants of ill health, there came a decline in 'crisis medicine' and the rise of a different form of intervention through public health. Here the emphasis was on prevention rather than cure (McKeown 1979). Public health, however, brought its own dilemmas; despite recognizing environmental determinants of ill health, it still strongly emphasized the importance of individual lifestyles. Further, although public health partly demystifies ill-health and prevention by emphasizing individual power over lifestyles, it also extends medicine's claims of competence to areas of personal and social life previously beyond its direct influence (Zola 1975). As we shall see, this extends to notions of appropriate behaviour on the part of individuals who are seeking, or 'should be' seeking, genetic services.

The dual themes of identification and cure, evident in scientific medicine and public health, could be seen to imply a concern with 'prevention' rather than 'informed decision-making'. The purpose of scientific medicine, and by association public health, is to create healthy people. This has become embodied in the professional activity of health professionals. The Royal College of Physicians (1989), in a report on genetic services, implicitly supports these assumptions by regarding the birth of a child with a genetic disorder as a medical failure. However, such ideas are influenced by other concerns that emphasize the importance of choice thus creating unresolvable tensions (Clarke 1991). These may include medico-legal issues that have occurred in the United States with, for example the threat of couples suing the health professionals for 'wrongful birth' (see Reilly 1992).

The idea of informed decision-making, however, is not entirely lost in the new genetics due to the powerful influence of liberal humanist thinking in the organization of western industrial societies, although this in turn can introduce ideas of prevention. Health care, including scientific medicine and public health, are influenced by a particular form of humanism associated with post-enlightenment thought. This form of humanism provides the West with its ideas of individualism, choice and emancipation. In particular, it offers a philosophy of action which maintains that individuals in pursuit of their own ends make their own history (Sopher 1986). People therefore have control over their own lives and require information to make informed decisions, enabling them to realize their ambitions. The 'new genetics' cannot be divorced from these discursive practices and they, in part, explain the emphasis on providing genetic information to enable 'informed decision-making' on the part of potential carriers. As we shall see, the wider context of citizenship and consumerism is central to such concerns.

At the same time, however, the influence of humanist philosophy contains contradictory elements that can be seen to support the idea of prevention and thus supporting the role of 'scientific medicine' (see Foucault 1977). In determining the rights of the citizens, new and extended patterns of surveillance are required. Scientific medicine and public health can be seen as part of this process. Humanist discourse, for example, lays down minimal requirements that identify human satisfaction and well being. In the absence of these requirements the individual is assumed 'unwell' and the conditions become the target of problem solving strategies. Alongside an apparent concern for others, individuals are 'monitored' to evaluate their functioning (Atkin 1991). Classification assumes great importance as a means to root out deviance and reform individuals. The 'new genetics', by drawing on the social practices of scientific medicine, partly supports this position. Identifying genetic conditions enables their prevention and this can be seen as a way of improving the human condition. However in doing so it creates potential for 'deviance' which then has to be corrected, something which, at its most extreme, has parallels with the eugenics project.

The concern to avoid possible eugenic connotation in the 'new genetics' is deeply embedded in the consciousness of present-day western industrial societies. Little more than 50 years ago National Socialist Germany, seeking to preserve the supposed superiority and purity of the Aryan 'race', committed the mass extermination of Jews, other minority ethnic groups, disabled people and 'social undesirables'. The implications of the World War II Holocaust raised uncertainty about eugenic thinking and its role in so-called 'civilized' societies (Harper 1992; Kevles 1999). Although the Holocaust represents the worst excesses of the eugenics project, both Britain and the USA have a strong history of eugenic thinking, a movement dating back to Galton and resulting in the formation of the Eugenics Education Society in 1907, which boasted membership of such luminaries as George

Bernard Shaw, the Webbs, J. Maynard Keynes, William Beveridge and Dr Barnardo (Williams 1996). The Eugenics Education Society was not a fringe group, but was a reflection of how seriously eugenic thinking was taken. The aim was to improve the human stock, encouraging the reproduction of those held to be superior and discouraging those believed to be inferior (Marteau and Richards 1996). The idea was that people should behave in a socially responsible way. Consequently, during the early part of the last century, eugenics became a potent force in social legislation in many industrial societies (Thom and Jennings 1996). The concern with social problems of the 1920s and 1930s, such as unemployment, pauperism, alcoholism and the supposed decline of the nations, found expression in the eugenic policies of population control.

The subsequent discrediting of eugenic thinking has meant it has had limited impact on haemoglobinopathies services in the UK. The spectre of eugenics tends to enforce the importance of informed decision-making rather than prevention controlled by professionals (Kevles 1999). This is an especially important dimension of providing screening for haemoglobinopathies because, in the UK sickle cell and thalassaemia occur largely in minority ethnic groups. Insensitive and top–down attempts at prevention therefore can be equated with the idea of eugenics. Presumed eugenicist overtones undermined the effectiveness of the first screening programmes established in the USA during the early 1970s. For example, the public recognition of sickle cell disorders in the USA was accompanied by the suggestion that the existence of sickle cell among African-Americans proved their genetic inferiority (Dyson 1998). Moreover, the emphasis on mass screening in many states seemed to focus explicitly on one disadvantaged ethnic minority group and could be regarded as an extension of state surveillance of black families (Bradby 1996). Bowman and Murray (1990: 126), two African-American doctors actively involved in genetic counselling in the USA, conclude:

> The legacy of National Socialism in Nazi Germany and of the eugenics movement in the United States necessitates caution in the enactment of genetics programs among minority ethnic groups, who may view efforts at prenatal diagnosis with selective abortion of affected fetuses as subtle genocide. This is particularly true if minority groups are poor, undernourished and undereducated and have high infant mortality rates, and if there is little prospect for change.

The idea of state surveillance is a particularly sensitive area in the UK because minority ethnic people are more likely to receive the controlling rather than the 'caring' aspect of state welfare (Atkin and Rollings 1993). Examples include black people's relationship with psychiatry (Sashidharan and Francis 1993), and the emphasis on birth control and the use of long-term contraceptives for black women (Williams 1996). To further illustrate this, Bhopal and White note the tendency of health professionals and researchers to concentrate on 'ethnic diseases' or problems, including fertility control in Britain, while 'an epidemic of coronary heart disease was sweeping through the South Asian community' (1993: 5). More generally, historical precedence, demonstrating the abuse of theories of inheritance, raises the possibility of racism in the development of the 'new genetics' (Bradby 1996; Dyson 1998). Identification of genetic conditions cannot be divorced from the previous racist practices experienced by minority groups (Atkin and Ahmad 1997). The symbolic association between genetic screening programmes and eugenics is perhaps unfortunate but nonetheless one that had a great impact on the consciousness of white liberals and African-Americans. Although African-Americans initially welcomed the sickle cell screening programmes as an initiative to meet their long neglected health care needs and as a means of controlling their own lives, the USA programme was subsequently described as racist (Bradby 1996). Subsequent debates mean that American screening programmes now have a greater emphasis on voluntary participation and informed decision-making (Loader *et al.* 1991).

The UK seemed to have learnt from these mistakes (Franklin 1990), hence the explicit emphasis on voluntary participation and informed decision-making in genetic screening programmes for haemoglobinopathies (Department of Health 1993). Haemoglobinopathy screening in pregnancy has however tended to become routinized with all the inherent hazards of assumed consent (Nuffield Council on Bioethics 1993). In this respect, the dangers of the ideology behind the eugenics movement are recognized and safeguards against it become an important organizing principle of genetic services (Bodmer and McKie 1994). Nonetheless ideas about 'genetic fitness' still occasionally occur when discussing 'humane' approaches to screening (see Modell and Kuliev 1991). More generally, as we will discuss, the informal culture of the health services broadly, as well as in genetic services, allows considerable discretion to individual professionals whose own racialized perspectives do influence the nature of service provision to minority ethnic people. Stereotypical assumptions about various ethnic groups, negative judgements and sweeping statements about the genetic consequences of first-cousin marriages, racist attitudes and inequitable access to specialist services can influence fears of a subtle eugenic agenda (Petrou *et al.* 1990).

Finally, this rather confused debate is also beginning to be informed by concepts of consumerism and citizenship. At a theoretical level, postmodern accounts, for example, point to the shift from production to consumption as a key organizing principle of western capitalism; the position once assumed by work has been replaced by the power of the consumer (Bauman 1992). Individuals thus seek to express themselves as free consumers exercising choice (Giddens 1991). Bauman argues that consumer conduct is moving steadily into the position of the cognitive and moral focus of life, the integrative bond of society, and the focus of systematic management.

These concerns with consumerism have also had a more practical focus. Policy changes in the organization and delivery of UK health and social care recognize both the role of citizenship and consumerism in achieving choice (see Plant *et al.* 1989). The old bureaucratic and paternalistic forms of public service where production and allocation are mediated by 'experts' – such as professionals, managers and administrators – have been undermined. Emerging out of these changes is a particular concern with 'getting close to the service user' and in particular the redistribution of power between health professionals and the individual (Hogg 1999).

The emphasis on the 'user' would enforce the principles of informed decision-making. In particular the state is seen as having a collective duty to ensure people's rights to be informed and to choose for themselves. This again would seem to enforce the idea of informed decision-making as a citizen's right (see Hogg 1999). In the UK, the demand for genetic testing for haemoglobinopathies often comes from minority ethnic communities themselves. This is often supported by white liberals. Prenatal diagnosis for thalassaemia, for instance, is often justified on the ground that the illness is a debilitating, life threatening condition with poor prospects for employment and career development (Ostrowsky *et al.* 1985). Such an approach emphasizes the right minority ethnic people have to be informed about their own lives, and as such, services for haemoglobinopathies represent a major site of struggle for ethnic minorities. As we have seen in the opening chapter, such support is often seen as a benchmark to assess the willingness and ability of the NHS to respond to the needs of ethnic minorities more generally (McNaught 1987).

Current changes in the management of welfare provision also mean the demand for genetic information could be seen in terms of consumer rights, where genetic information can become a basis of constructing self-image and life choices. Genetic testing kits, for instance, could become as popular as home pregnancy kits. Already it is possible, for example, to purchase mail order kits that determine whether an individual is a carrier of cystic fibrosis. Further, a gene 'shop' was opened at Manchester Airport for one year, from February 1997–98. The shop, offering advice and information on a variety of genetic disorders, was modelled on the Citizen's Advice Bureaux with the hope of attracting passers-by who wished to know more about genetic disorders. The consumer emphasis on individual choice could have empowering consequences and create the demand for genetic information as the basis of informed decision-making. According to Levitt (2000: 77), however,

> the Gene Shop could be seen as a success when evaluated in terms of its stated aims but it embodied a deficit model of public understanding with content which portrayed developments in the science of genetics and its applications as an unproblematic progression.

However, popular conceptions of citizenship are characterized as much by rights as by duties (Flynn 1989). Social and economic rights to collective resources do not exist outside an obligation to society as a whole; citizenship rights are conditional on the discharge of obligations (Mead 1986). Potentially this approach to citizenship has important implications for genetic information. As we have seen, humanist philosophy and notions such as consumerism can emphasize the importance of informed decision-making in dealing with genetic conditions. Aspects of citizenship enforce this. Citizenship rights, on the other hand, might also imply the responsible use of genetic information and compliance with medical advice (Green 1993).

From an international perspective, who should determine what should be perceived as morally right for any particular society? In an anonymized questionnaire survey of Chinese geneticists, of whom 255 out of 402 (63 per cent) responded, 91 per cent thought that couples who find that they are both carriers should not proceed to have children together and 91 per cent thought that women should have a prenatal diagnosis if medically indicated (Mao 1998). Marteau *et al.* (1994) compared how geneticists in Germany, Portugal and the UK reported counselling women following diagnosis of a fetus, for one of a range of conditions. Despite strong professional codes of non-directiveness, geneticists report being somewhat directive in some counselling situations. German and Portuguese geneticists, in different ways, were significantly more directive than UK geneticists with German geneticists more likely to encourage continuation of pregnancies, while those from Portugal were more likely to encourage termination of affected pregnancies.

This issue raises important dilemmas. If a person reasonably suspects that they could carry a genetic condition do they have a responsibility to be tested? If he or she is likely to give birth to an affected child should they, as responsible citizens, abort the affected child? Does their non-compliance or refusal to abort shift them into the category of the undeserving in terms of access to state welfare? If they do not choose abortion should they then be responsible for the costs of bringing up the affected child? We, of course, do not suggest these are legitimate questions. Nonetheless, they can easily emerge and responding to them is far from straightforward, as debate can become corrupted with an emphasis on responsibility and an individualistic conception of citizenship which emphasizes responsibilities of citizens as much as it underplays their rights.

Organizing haemoglobinopathy screening services

Besides the philosophical concerns discussed above, there are more practical aspects of providing screening and counselling services for haemoglobinopathies. Exploring these practical aspects begins to explain the difficulties faced by those at risk of haemoglobinopathies as well as identify potential sites of strategy and struggle for those wishing to improve services. Various issues emerge and these include the meaning of screening and counselling for the general population; the psychological and social implications for people identified as carriers; the process of providing information to carriers; and the organization and delivery of services. Each of these issues, unable to transcend the tension between informed decision-making and prevention, illustrates the difficulties of establishing screening for SCD and thalassaemia and perhaps contributes to the poor coordination of provision in the UK (Department of Health 1993).

The meaning of screening and counselling for the lay population

There is an emerging literature on the general meaning ascribed to screening and counselling for genetic conditions by the lay population. As we have seen, screening for recessive conditions such as haemoglobinopathies is often ad hoc. Practitioners, for example, often guess a person's ethnic origin when deciding whom to test (Anionwu 1993; Atkin *et al.* 1998a, 1998b; Bain and Chapman 1998; Dyson 1999). In other cases, whether a person is tested or not depends on the knowledge of the health professional with whom they have contact (Atkin *et al.* 1998a, 1998b). Further, counselling can be offered by a range of practitioners, ranging from specialist haemoglobinopathy counsellors to consultant physicians (Department of Health 1993; Zeuner *et al.* 1999). Consequently, there is no consistent model for either screening or counselling (Modell and Anionwu 1996). This begins to introduce an element of confusion into the lay population's understanding.

More generally, much of the empirical evidence on people's response to genetic screening and counselling is based on the experience of white populations. The sparse literature on the experience of minority ethnic communities, however, illustrates both differences and similarities with the broader literature. In the first instance, most people are positive about the development of genetic screening and only about 1 in 50 say they would not want to be screened for genetic conditions (Green and Statham 1996). However the take-up of genetic screening services for both dominant and recessive conditions does not seem to match people's expressed enthusiasm for such tests (Richards 1993; Hill 1994). How then do people come forward for genetic testing?

Genetic screening is often presented, along with other testing, as part of an antenatal package. For many people, especially women, this represents their first and only contact with genetic screening services. Mothers, however, are often not aware of the array of tests to which they are subject, and seem to accept the testing of themselves and the unborn child uncritically (Firdous and Bhopal 1989; Richards and Green 1993). Mothers' knowledge of screening tests for which they are eligible and which they may have undergone is frequently low (Marteau *et al.* 1992), and especially low for minority ethnic women (Firdous and Bhopal 1989). Consequently, mothers accept rather than explicitly consent to such tests, which are seen as a taken-for-granted aspect of antenatal care, without always appreciating the potential consequences of screening (Richards 1993). These assumptions are shared by health professionals who rarely explain the nature and consequences of such tests to the mother (Green and Statham 1996). In many cases, little information is given about testing, the conditions screened for, and the meaning of either a positive or a negative result (Marteau *et al.* 1992). Evidence even suggest that some pregnant women have never been informed that their blood samples would be screened for haemoglobin-opathies (Black and Laws 1986; Anionwu *et al.* 1988; Eboh and van den Akker 1995). Often only if a mother objects to such a test is she offered genetic counselling (Green and Statham 1996). One potential consequence of these findings would be that the relatively more compliant behaviour of minority women (Bhopal and White 1993), would lead to greater acceptance of medical advice and testing. Indeed this is the case for immunizations where minority ethnic communities have higher rates of immunization than the white population (Baker *et al.* 1984).

Presentation of genetic testing as a routine part of antenatal care is further reflected in the mother's relationship with maternity services (Pembrey and Anionwu 1996). Mothers often perceive genetic testing as a way of ensuring normality rather than detecting abnormality (Richards 1993). For example, those who say they would not accept termination may quite rationally judge this to be irrelevant to their decision to accept screening (Green and Statham 1996). In the case of the genetic disorder being detected some couples may have already firmly decided whether or not to terminate the pregnancy (Chitty *et al.* 1996). In this respect there seems to be a fundamental difference of opinion between obstetricians and mothers (Rothman 1993). Obstetricians put the emphasis on detection of abnormalities, whereas mothers are seeking reassurance that all is well (Richards and Green 1993). This is an issue we return to later in the chapter.

The emphasis on testing during pregnancy raises another important aspect of the debate: the gendered nature of identifying recessive conditions (Shiloh 1996). The new genetics alters the way in which pregnancy and childbirth are understood. For example, Stacey (1996) observes that the focus is on producing a 'healthy baby' rather than the woman carrying the child. However, women assume a key role in receiving and then disseminating genetic knowledge. It is usually the woman who has to negotiate with the health professional on the basis of what she has understood, and then negotiate with her partner, family and kin about the significance of such information (Stacey 1996). Work on haemoglobinopathies supports this (Atkin *et al.* 1998b).

More general interest in carrier detection is limited because most people who have not had direct contact do not see themselves as being at risk of genetic conditions (Richards and Green 1993). One possible explanation is that individuals hold views about inheritance suggesting they cannot be a carrier if they do not have a close relative with the disease (Richards and Green 1993). The belief of not being prone to the disease or being a carrier is indicated by the low take-up of screening for cystic fibrosis (Richards 1993) and leads to shock and disbelief when carriers have been found in cystic fibrosis programmes (Watson *et al.* 1992). Similar findings have been reported for haemoglobinopathy screening in the USA (Hill 1994).

Understanding and knowledge seems to be an important influence on the take-up of genetic services. Certainly in Cyprus, there is a high up-take of screening services for thalassaemia. The widespread experiences of caring for a person with thalassaemia and the accompanying financial and emotional stresses are often associated with the success of the thalassaemia screening programme in Cyprus (Richards 1993; Bradby 1996). This is not to say that screening is not without its problems and a degree of stigma is still associated with carrier status (Anionwu 1993). Nonetheless, debates about screening have become located within wider civil society and are not solely associated with state imposition (Angastiniotis *et al.* 1986). The Greek Orthodox Church, for example, will refuse to marry a couple unless they show evidence that they have been screened for thalassaemia at an authorized centre (Marteau and Anionwu 1996). Cypriot communities in Britain have a similarly high take-up of screening services. Indeed the use of carrier detection in combination with fetal diagnosis and abortion have more or less eliminated births of children with thalassaemia major in the British Cypriot communities (Gill and Modell 1999). However this response to thalassaemia seems different to that of Asian communities living in the UK. Compared to countries such as Italy, Greece and Cyprus, the UK has the lowest fall in births of children affected with thalassaemia and is largely attributed to births to Asian communities, particularly British Pakistanis (Modell and Kuliev 1992; Gill and Modell 1999).

The reasons for this are complex and relatively unexplored. Nor, as we have argued above, should the lack of success in reducing the number of births among Asian communities be seen as a failure. Nonetheless, various reasons help us make sense of this difference between ethnic groups. As we have argued, dealing with thalassaemia has not become part of the cultural repertoire of the Asian communities as it is among people from Greece and Cyprus (Dyson *et al.* 1993). Discussion about the issue, for instance, has been rare among Asian communities. Differences in knowledge of genetic conditions are perhaps all-important. A national survey undertaken by the UK Thalassaemia Society in 1996 identified that only 5 per cent of Asian people had heard of thalassaemia (Lakhani 1999). Equally we must also explore further the factors relating to the organization of services (Modell *et al.* 2000a) and in particular the consequences of racist assumptions (Dyson 1998; Darr 1999). As we shall see, abortion is assumed to be unacceptable to Asian people and therefore not always offered as an option (Atkin *et al.* 1998b). This runs contrary to evidence suggesting that attitudes towards abortion among South Asian groups, are fluid across and within families as well as for individuals over different pregnancies (Darr 1990; Atkin *et al.* 1998a, 1998b). This is an issue we return to later in the chapter when we discuss the diagnosis of haemoglobinopathies.

On the other hand African-Caribbean communities usually acknowledge sickle cell disorders as an important condition. Haemoglobinopathy services represent a particular site of struggle for African-Caribbean communities and evidence suggests a somewhat better, although still superficial, knowledge of sickle cell among these groups than knowledge of thalassaemia among Asian people (Anionwu 1993; Dyson *et al*. 1993; Dyson 1997, Green and France-Dawson 1997; Lakhani 1999). Consequently sickle cell disorders and struggles around its official recognition have become an important element of African-Caribbean identity and engagement with the state. African-Caribbean people's response to sickle cell supports this (Atkin *et al*. 2000). Young people with SCD, for instance, are more likely to associate their condition with 'black' identity than those with thalassaemia (Atkin and Ahmad 1997). Nonetheless, African-Caribbean people still only have a limited understanding of sickle cell and thalassaemia, of conditions for which tests are available during the antenatal period, and more generally about genetically inherited diseases. In a study by Green and France-Dawson (1997) virtually all (98 per cent) African-Caribbean respondents had heard of SCD. Closer examination, however, suggested important misunderstandings. For example, 38 per cent understood sickle cell trait to be a milder form of the disease.

More generally, it is important not to confuse greater awareness and improved service provision with a greater willingness to accept termination of affected children. Greater understanding and improved provision should be a goal in its own right. Further, acknowledgement is needed for difference in attitudes towards prenatal diagnosis and abortion. Several studies reveal, for example, that around 30 per cent of women – irrespective of ethnicity – would not consider termination on the grounds of fetal abnormality (Green and Statham 1996). Service provision should perhaps accept this rather than see it as a failure of communication (Atkin and Ahmad 1997). Decision-making of this kind is a much more complex process for ethnic minorities, who are dominated numerically, economically and politically by a predominately white and ethnocentric society (Bradby 1996; Dyson 1997).

Before leaving our discussion of the knowledge of screening and counselling, it is also necessary to emphasize that sickle cell and thalassaemia, like many other conditions, have a social dimension. There is a considerable body of literature describing how the social meaning of disability and the disadvantages that occur is as much a limitation on the lives of disabled people as their physical impairment (Oliver 1996; Shakespeare 1999 and Chapter 5 explore these issues in greater detail). Clarke (1991) makes the observation that some older people's support for euthanasia could derive from social pressure that constructs them as a 'burden'. The choice made by parents in aborting an affected child is, therefore, influenced by socialization, perceived or experienced social pressures, as well as concerns about the medical outcome of the condition. Although screening is purportedly about offering an informed choice, nonetheless it is impossible to avoid the normative implicit assumption about the undesirability of the existence of people with such a condition and of giving birth to and bringing up such people (Stacey 1996). The promotion of screening programmes cannot help but carry a moral message about the worth of the lives of those individuals who have these disorders (Clarke 1991). In response to this, Shakespeare (1999) highlights the absence of a disability perspective in research on the cultural construction of genetics and argues the need for a greater dialogue between the medical establishment and the civil rights movement of disabled people. In this respect, deafness provides an interesting example. To counter increased interest in the prenatal diagnosis of deafness, some deaf individuals have argued – perhaps polemically – for the right to terminate non-deaf children.

The social aspects of screening mean that parents have to weigh up various considerations in reaching a decision on the testing or continuation of a pregnancy (Rothman 1993). Do the parents feel they have sufficient resources to care for an affected child? How are their decisions affected by the prevalent medical discourses? How does the wider society treat disabled people? How will their family and wider community react to the birth of an affected child or the decision to terminate? What impact will the decision have on the person's personal, moral, gender or religious identity? A case study presented by Atkin *et al.* (1998b) shows that one of the mothers in their research decided to terminate a child affected by thalassaemia on the basis of how the wider society would treat a person with a chronic illness, rather than on the severity of the illness. Much of the disadvantage and discrimination faced by those with a haemoglobinopathy is socially constructed and a consequence of society's difficulty to accommodate those who are in any way 'different'. The next chapter illustrates how this becomes a defining aspect informing the experience of those with a haemoglobinopathy and their families.

The process of providing information on genetic testing

Another practical difficulty in organizing haemoglobinopathy services is the process of providing information. We touched on this above and suggested that a fundamental problem was the mismatch between ideas held by health professionals who provide testing and counselling and the users (Rapp 1988). The understanding may be even more limited where there is a language or cultural gap between service providers and parents, issues considered later in the chapter. Generally, individuals do not make simple choices in light of relevant information; a variety of personal and social factors influence decisions (Michie and Marteau 1996). For instance, most at-risk parents' general understanding, although complex, does not mirror formal discourse on genetics (Atkin *et al.* 1998b). Those providing information often fail to recognize this, while at the same time pursuing their own agendas without reference to the patients' concerns. For example in one study, 58 per cent of US genetic counsellors were not aware of the topic the counsellees wanted to discuss (Wertz *et al.* 1986).

In some respects the process of providing information is confused by the tension between prevention and informed decision-making. As we have discussed, obstetricians are motivated by the concerns to eliminate 'abnormality' rather than necessarily broadening choice while mothers seek confirmation of 'normality' (Marteau and Richards 1996; Atkin *et al.* 1998b). Atkin *et al.* (1998b) note that some consultants, for example, assume that if a woman suspected of carrying a child with thalassaemia major received a positive prenatal test, she would automatically abort the fetus. Consultants felt that by agreeing to take the test, the parents had tacitly agreed to an abortion if the result was positive. Since the test carried a small risk to the fetus and was expensive, any other option was deemed unreasonable. That the parents may wish to use the test to arrive at an informed decision, which includes the possibility of rejecting medical advice, did not appear to be a legitimate position to these consultants. Other work confirms this directive approach (Farrant 1980). For example, 75 per cent of obstetricians suggest that the patient agree to the termination of an affected pregnancy before proceeding with amniocentesis or chorionic villus sampling (Green 1993). More generally, many consultants, drawing on their professional socialization, have few problems in advocating termination of affected children, especially in thalassaemia (Atkin *et al.* 1998b). This exercise of power denies knowledge and choice to parents who do not wish to choose abortion (Stacey 1996).

These problems are further exacerbated by the discretionary nature of counselling provision (Wertz *et al.* 1990). The actual process of genetic counselling usually takes place behind closed doors and has, until recently, been subject to little observation, monitoring or audit. It is therefore difficult to assess the degree to which a stated objective is actually achieved in practice. Findings from various studies, for example, reveal directiveness on consultations by those who perceive themselves as being non-directive (Rothman 1988; Michie *et al.* 1997). Moreover, within the NHS, there are no defined models of counselling. Although some localities employ specialist haemoglobinopathy counsellors, counselling and disclosure are often undertaken by health professionals with little formal training in counselling, limited understanding of users' cultural backgrounds, and often through poorly trained interpreters or family members (Atkin *et al.* 1998b). Thus many parents are denied specialist support and informed choice.

Further, an understanding of the process of information exchange in genetic counselling is not straightforward. Individuals do not make simple choices in light of relevant information, and where they are steered towards certain decisions, this steering can be imperceptible (Atkin and Ahmad 1997). As we have seen, when screening is offered, it is difficult to avoid the message that the disorder in question is serious enough to justify termination of the pregnancy (Clarke 1991). Those offered these tests probably know little about the disorder they are being invited to avoid. Therefore, the implicit message might be unduly influential (Green and Statham 1996; see also above).

More practically, people do not understand genetic information in the way intended by health professionals (Atkin *et al.* 1998b). This may have nothing to do with intellectual or emotional difficulties but result from a different conception of genetic knowledge (Richards and Green 1993). Lay perceptions of inheritance, genes, risk and prevention differ markedly from professional perceptions (Rapp 1988). In the case of cystic fibrosis, for example, carriers may not accept it as a 'genetic condition' but still hold it runs in families (Richards 1993). Nor are ideas of risk uniform; statistical risk is not always easily accommodated in lay knowledge, and concepts such as 'fairness' also come into play. Some parents, for example, interpreted a one-in-four risk of having a child with SCD as high; others regard it as low (Atkin *et al.* 1998b). The same research also illustrates that parents who already have a child with a haemoglobinopathy believe the next three pregnancies will produce a child without the condition (Atkin *et al.* 1998b).

The notion that a healthy individual (a carrier) can pass on a genetic disease is also questioned by parents (Atkin *et al.* 1998b). Holding such a view has little to do with denial but is a common-sense application of personal knowledge of the social world (Michie and Marteau 1996). Such world views can tolerate ambiguities and contradictions. Counsellors, on the other hand, may hold that problems can be overcome, but pre-existing beliefs may prevent families from understanding or acting on information. The health professional is not simply a neutral provider of information. Their location within a culturally specific, professionally produced structure is important in understanding the interface between lay public and genetic services (Atkin and Ahmad 1997).

When a gap exists between the attitudes and expectation of health care professionals and patients, there is a tendency to try and bridge this gap by inducing patients to conform to the view of health care professionals (Hill 1994). For these reasons Richards (1993) concludes that the non-directive emphasis in counselling is understandable, but does not provide a very helpful starting point for the discussion of genetic counselling which by its nature and location within biomedicine constructs certain choices as the 'common-sense' choices, particularly since evidence suggests that health service provision ignores lay people's understanding of their health (Turner 1989). There is often conflict between the lay logic and that promoted by professionals, with the patient or client viewpoint subordinated to the professional view (Stimson and Webb 1975). As Rapp (1988) observes, the language of biomedical science is powerful, although appearing neutral and non-judgemental. However the medical discourse creates a tension between the universal abstract language of reproductive medicine, and the personal experiences articulated by women (Rapp 1988). Medical knowledge commands great authority but cannot always respond to all questions women bring to the encounter. Despite counsellors' attempts to adjust to patient's language, the emerging language difficulties may signal communicative ambiguities far beyond the question of literal translation. In effect local metaphors do not easily translate into medical discourse (Rapp 1988). Hill (1994), for example, illustrates how women actively reinterpreted medical information on SCD so that it accorded with their own beliefs and experiences.

Such gaps in understanding between professionals and patients may be greater where information exchange takes place across cultural and linguistic divides (Anionwu 1996b) and when power differences between professionals and clients also reflect historical relations of racial exploitation and subordination. Racism, for instance, is a particular influence in the development of haemoglobinopathy provision (Ahmad 1993) and is a core theme of this book.

Professionals' assumptions about South Asian patients' refusal to terminate affected pregnancies, as we have seen, led to the denial of choice to many Asian parents, thus reflecting the role of cultural myths in undermining accepted good practice (Department of Health 1993; Ahmad and Atkin 1996a). Abortions, for a variety of reasons, are carried out by both medical as well as traditional practitioners in Pakistan, India and Bangladesh, so the idea of selective abortion is not entirely alien to the British Asians. Further, South Asian people's responses to termination are as variable and complex as any other section of the population (Green 1992). Termination was acceptable to some families but not to others and further, that some parents may make different decisions during different pregnancies (Darr 1990; Atkin *et al.* 1998b). The organization of services further undermines the choice offered to Asian families. Many Asian women come into antenatal care later than their white counterparts – a phenomenon more related to the quality of general practitioner care than the individual 'failings' of Asian women (Clarke and Clayton 1983) – and therefore any 'abnormality' is more likely to be detected in the second trimester when termination is less acceptable to women (Parsons *et al.* 1993). Indeed the most common reason, among Asian families, for turning down prenatal diagnosis was the timing of the test, often during the second trimester (Modell *et al.* 2000a) and to this extent they are perhaps no different from the general population (Richards 1993). Consequently, there are a series of psychological and emotional, as well as social and moral reasons why an abortion at an advanced stage will be unacceptable and this applies equally to white women. Yet many practitioners falsely attributed Asian families' reluctance to accept prenatal diagnosis to religious objections to termination (Atkin *et al.* 1998b).

The social and psychological consequences of identifying people as carriers

Some authors have suggested that carrier status for genetic conditions may constitute a spoiled identity which becomes especially salient at particular times in the life cycle, such as the early stages of a new relationship, marriage, or when planning a pregnancy (Parsons and Atkinson 1992). There is little research assessing the consequences of people's responses to such damaged identity, and the impact is likely to be context specific (Atkin and Ahmad 1997). Identification of carriers raises the obvious dilemma between increasing people's control over their own lives and the incumbent psychological burden of such knowledge (Shiloh 1996). In some communities and other conditions, consequences may be considerable. For Tay Sachs disease, for example, there is some evidence that carriers find it difficult to find marriage partners (Parsons and Atkinson 1992). Further, as a consequence of a screening programme in a Greek village, carriers were socially neglected by those who were non-carriers (McKie 1988). There is evidence that some professionals as well as employers and insurance companies interpret the trait as a milder form of the condition, which may have consequences for employment (Franklin and Atkin 1986). Evidence from a study examining the psychological and social consequences of community carrier screening programmes for cystic fibrosis revealed that anxiety associated initially with a positive result could be allayed by genetic counselling (Watson *et al.* 1992). Although we do not have much published evidence on thalassaemia in this respect, personal testimonials from people with the condition at the Thalassaemia Society's annual conference recount many stories of relational difficulties, problems in securing employment, and difficulties in securing mortgages and insurance. This is certainly a feature of parents and young people's narratives (Atkin and Ahmad 1997; Atkin *et al.* 2000).

Policy in screening for haemoglobinopathies, however, creates the danger of separating the counselling and screening; this split will become greater with the possible introduction of genetic testing kits – currently for cystic fibrosis – available through mail order (see above). Accessibility of such kits creates an interesting tension; on the one hand it breaks the monopoly of the medical profession on screening and thus gives power to the consumer, but on the other hand it distances screening even more from counselling. The former Advisory Committee on Genetic Testing (now superseded by the Human Genetics Commission) addressed these concerns by producing a Code of Practice (1997). The connection between screening and counselling, however, is not always straightforward and can raise fundamental ethical dilemmas. Some areas now screen newborn babies for haemoglobinopathies. Screening tests not only identify those with the condition, but also carriers. Should parents be informed that their newborn child is a carrier of sickle cell, even though that information is of no immediate use and is potentially anxiety-provoking? At the same time is it right to withhold such information from parents? Finally, who has the right to this information anyway, the parent or the child? There is no clear policy guidance on these issues (Laird *et al.* 1996).

Diagnosing sickle cell and thalassaemia: policy and practice

The process of telling parents that their child has been born with SCD or thalassaemia reflects many of the problems described above. Racialized assumptions as well as differences of opinion between parents and health professionals are commonplace (Atkin *et al.* 1998a, 1998b). The long-term neglect of these conditions by the NHS which results in poor service coordination and low priority given to haemoglobinopathies is also evident (Anionwu 1993). Families, therefore, often receive inadequate support during diagnosis (Atkin *et al.* 1998a).

Diagnosis is a key period for parents of a child with a chronic illness (Eiser 1990). Early diagnosis enhances the prospects for adequate care, adjustment and coping (Sloper and Turner 1992; Beresford 1996a). A study by Hall *et al.* (2000) on the psychological impact on parents of children with Down's syndrome following either a false negative result or a failure to offer screening, cites the range of evidence that blaming others is associated with poor adjustment to a wide range of negative events. Awaiting a diagnosis is also a time of distress and uncertainty (Green and Statham 1996), evoking feelings of guilt, frustration, anxiety, helplessness and resentment (Atkin 1992), particularly since parents usually anticipate a 'healthy' child (Richards 1993). Diagnosing haemoglobinopathies raises specific difficulties for parents (Department of Health 1993; Modell and Anionwu 1996). Early diagnosis, as we have seen, is essential. Without diagnosis and treatment thalassaemics die before the age of 2, and up to 30 per cent of deaths in SCD occur before diagnosis (Midence and Elander 1994). However, the experience of parents – especially those whose child has an SCD – suggests that diagnosis of haemoglobinopathies is unpredictable (Atkin and Ahmad 2000a).

Formal policy and practice confirms parents' experience (Department of Health 1993). Few localities, for example, operate a universal screening policy (Health Education Authority 1998). Selective policies were justified on the grounds of the small at-risk populations and limited resources (Modell and Anionwu 1996). Consequently, it is rare for NHS Trusts to operate a coherent policy; in most cases, ethnic stereotypes drove screening policy whereby parents were selected on the basis of ethnicity as judged by skin colour or name (Atkin *et al.* 1998b). Not surprisingly, carriers were often not identified and conditions sometimes misdiagnosed if the person did not fit these ethnic stereotypes of at-risk groups. A survey of UK antenatal screening practice by Bain and Chapman (1998) revealed that out of 38 localities involved in selective screening only 23 requested information on ethnic origin. Of these only four received this information on request forms for more than 20 per cent of patients. District Health Authorities often add to the confusion by not knowing about the activities of NHS Trusts to steer policy and practice (Streetly *et al.* 1997; Atkin *et al.* 1998b), a problem also noted in other areas of the NHS (Flynn *et al.* 1996).

The role of primary health care further complicates the process (Modell *et al.* 1998). Primary health care is seen as being at the forefront of the new NHS (Department of Health 1997). As a reflection of this, the role of primary health care workers in providing haemoglobinopathy screening is advocated by various policy documents (Department of Health 1993; Health Education Authority 1998). Evidence suggests, however, that primary health care is not an ideal basis for screening provision but there are notable exceptions (Ahmad and Atkin 2000). Logan (2000) has argued that haemoglobinopathy screening can be undertaken in primary care and describes the model developed in her own general practice in south London, which has been recognized by the NHS Executive as a beacon practice for this service. GPs, for example, are often criticized for not explaining the significance of test results to parents or not understanding test results themselves (Atkin *et al.* 1998b). Further, they often refer patients to hospital services too late for it be of value for screening and informed decisions by parents (Modell *et al.* 1998; Harris *et al.* 1999; Ahmad and Atkin 2000; Modell *et al.* 2000a). Other research supports this view, indicating insufficient monitoring of minority ethnic pregnant women in primary health care (Parsons *et al.* 1993), late referrals to hospital antenatal care (Jain 1985) and poor quality provision (Clarke and Clayton 1983). Moreover GPs may not fully understand the value and purpose of genetic testing (Royal College of Physicians 1989; Modell *et al.* 1998).

Another major problem is the lack of understanding among health professionals generally about the relevance of screening and diagnosis (Midence and Elander 1994; Anionwu 1996a). This is particularly significant given the discretionary nature of screening policy in many areas (see above). This lack of knowledge is also evident during diagnosis. Service managers and health commissioners, for example, are aware that basic presenting symptoms of the two conditions are sometimes missed by health professionals (Atkin *et al.* 1998b). Policy guidance on haemoglobinopathies supports this view (Davies *et al.* 1993; Department of Health 1993).

Provision of information and emotional support during diagnosis is also poor (Black and Laws 1986; Darr 1990), which can prolong uncertainty and potentially undermine a parent's ability to come to terms with the diagnosis (Turner and Sloper 1992). Diagnosing SCD seems especially problematic (Davies *et al.* 1993). Parents often experience lengthy periods of misdiagnosis (Midence and Elander 1994). To make the situation worse the legitimate concerns of parents are often disregarded and this is a particular problem for mothers who found themselves dismissed as 'neurotic' or 'overprotective' (Atkin *et al.* 1998b). These authors provide an example of one mother, whose concerns were regularly dismissed by health professionals. She was even given counselling support to help her overcome her 'morbid obsession' with her daughter's health. After five years of struggling to obtain a diagnosis, her daughter was diagnosed as having a SCD. Gender as well as ethnic stereotypes seem to explain these medical responses to parents' concerns (McIntyre and Oldham 1977; Beresford 1996a). Not surprisingly, many parents see diagnosis as something that had to be fought for (Hill 1994) and this is similar to accounts of diagnostic process in other genetic conditions (Green and Murton 1996).

This battle continues as the parents pursue information about the illness at the time of diagnosis (Atkin *et al.* 1998b). This is especially frustrating from the parents' point of view because general evidence suggests that appropriate information can facilitate successful coping (Baldwin and Carlisle 1994). People with SCD or thalassaemia, however, often complain about a lack of information and express doubts about the ability or willingness of health professionals to provide such information (Darr 1990; Midence and Elander 1994). Common complaints include confusing, inadequate or rushed explanations, lack of an opportunity to ask questions and a failure on the part of consultants to volunteer information (Atkin *et al.* 1998b). Parents, therefore, find it difficult to come to terms with the diagnosis, as well as being deprived of information that would help them care for their child. These problems seem common during the process of diagnosing childhood disability (Sloper and Turner 1992; Green and Murton 1996).

Despite these problems in diagnosing haemoglobinopathies, the rise of sickle cell and thalassaemia counsellors or specialist workers, whose employment was often secured as a consequence of community activity, has helped improve the sensitivity of provision in many areas (Streetly *et al.* 1997). The majority are minority ethnic nurses and midwives (Anionwu 1996b) and the importance of these workers in providing support to affected individuals and their families will be a recurring theme of this book. Parents and young people, for example, speak highly of these workers' involvement in their care (Atkin *et al.* 1998b). The process of diagnosis reflected this. Parents in contact with specialist workers, for example, felt the condition was well explained and found workers approachable (Atkin *et al.* 1998a; Atkin and Ahmad 2000a). Ongoing contact with these workers was particularly valued, particularly since parents did not regard a one-off information session as adequate. Emotional support provided by these workers was also highly valued by parents, who often welcomed the opportunity to talk through their shock, worries and concerns about having a chronically ill child. Another specific advantage of these specialist workers was that they shared their patients' linguistic and cultural background (Atkin *et al.* 2000). This is particularly important since the problems in obtaining information are compounded for those who could not speak or understand English. Language support is generally poor and as a consequence people from minority ethnic backgrounds are often denied important information about the illness (Butt 1994; Walker and Ahmad 1994). The issues raised by communication also emphasize the importance of recognizing cultural difference in providing support to those with the illness and their families, especially since most health professionals feel ill-equipped to respond to these differences (Bowler 1993). The issues of inadequate language support and recognizing cultural differences are discussed more fully in subsequent chapters.

Various tensions, however, still exist in the counsellors' role (Potrykus 1993). These counsellors cannot transcend the tensions between 'informed decision-making' and 'prevention'. Two factors might be important in generating witting or unwitting pressure on counsellors. The first are the differences in uptake of prenatal diagnosis and termination of pregnancies by those at risk of children with SCD compared to those at risk of children with beta thalassaemia major. An example of this is noted in the HTA review by Davies *et al.* (2000) which reports that the data from Central

Middlesex Hospital in Brent found that 80 per cent of beta thalassaemia births and 16 per cent of sickle cell anaemia births were prevented by universal antenatal screening. They add: 'it is likely therefore that previous British studies have overestimated the impact of universal antenatal screening in preventing SCD births' (Davies *et al*. 2000: iv). The second concern is when there is a temptation to measure the effectiveness of sickle and thalassaemia counsellors by comparing uptake levels for prenatal diagnosis and terminations of affected pregnancies in women counselled by different practitioners. What unites these two issues is that there has been little research in the UK that, first, compares the views and experiences of a significant number of couples at risk of having children with the two disorders and, second, that observes the actual process of haemoglobinopathy counselling by specialist workers. In the absence of such studies stereotypical assumptions can too easily be made about the actions of at-risk couples together with negative aspersions concerning the 'effectiveness' of certain types of haemoglobinopathy screening and counselling. All of this reflects the tension between 'informed decision-making' and 'prevention' discussed above.

Conclusion

This chapter discusses screening and counselling for haemoglobinopathies within the broader context of the 'new genetics'. In doing so, it introduces key themes – such as equity, access and the value of political engagement – fundamental in making sense of the politics of sickle cell and thalassaemia. These themes, as we shall see, reoccur throughout the book. More specifically, this chapter identifies two concerns that currently inform shortfalls in screening and diagnosing those at risk of haemoglobinopathies.

First, the ideals of informed decision-making are not always adhered to in practice because of ideas about 'prevention'. The often racialized and stereotypical perspectives of service professionals further limit choice. These observations are not intended to undermine the provision of screening and counselling services. We are concerned, however, that prevention is not always driven by informed decision-making. Consequently, recognizing the various tensions in current provision can help inform more accessible and appropriate provision for those at risk of haemoglobinopathies. This is the basis of empowerment.

Second, the current state of screening and counselling provision rarely meets the needs of at-risk populations. Understanding the various problems provides an agenda for future activity to improve such provision. Policy and practice, therefore, needs to address the difficulties faced by families. These include the need to respect the concerns of parents and those with the illness, a coherent and comprehensive screening and counselling policy, improved training of frontline practitioners, and better provision of information.

More generally, poor quality care, inadequate information, insensitivity to the 'at-risk' families' worries and failure to meet their needs become central to our analysis. People's experiences of screening and diagnosis have parallels with the substantial literature on the difficulties minority ethnic people face in having their health care needs met, recognized and catered for (Ahmad and Atkin 1996a); especially since the inability to meet the linguist and cultural needs of affected groups characterize haemoglobinopathy provision for screening and diagnosis. Equally, parents' high regard for specialist workers reminds us that services can be sensitive and empowering. Good practice does exist and it is important that this informs future provision. The next two chapters develop these general ideas further.

Note

1 Some clinics, such as those offering genetic advice for those families who have inherited cancer, make no pretence of being non-directive. The tensions between informed decision-making and prevention is thus irrelevant. Recessive conditions, however, at least seem to offer people the opportunity to make informed reproductive choices.

5

The experience of sickle cell and thalassaemia

There was evidence that such patients [with sickle cell disorders and thalassaemia] are not always looked after in the best possible way, even in districts where these disorders are common.

(Department of Health 1993: 11)

The previous chapter focused on the difficulties faced by individuals and families during screening and diagnosis. This chapter begins to discuss the everyday experience of living with a sickle cell or thalassaemia disorder. It explores the difficulties faced by affected individuals and their families as well as the strategies adopted as people cope with the consequences of the two illnesses. Describing this experience is valid in its own right as it provides an insight into the lives of people with a haemoglobinopathy and their families (Midence and Elander 1994). Such a discussion also begins to identify legitimate areas of strategy and struggle, aimed at improving understanding and support.

Those with the illness have to face regular disruptions to their everyday lives because of the complications associated with their illness (Darr 1990; Anionwu 1993; Streetly *et al*. 1997; Maxwell *et al*. 1999; see also Chapters 2 and 3). These disruptions often challenge a person's self-identity, make social interaction perilous and potentially increase dependence on others (Midence and Elander 1994). Families may also face considerable difficulties as they offer care for a chronically ill member (Atkin *et al*. 1998a). Despite the impact of haemoglobinopathies on individuals, the intention, however, is not to present people and their families as tragic victims at the mercy of the illness. Rather, the chapter suggests that the affected people are active agents struggling against disadvantage and discrimination as well as balancing other competing social roles – such as employees, family members and friends – with having a chronic illness.

Empowerment must begin from this premise (Bourdieu 1984) and be further grounded in the broader economic, social and political context

(Harrison 1993). As an introduction to this, the experience of individuals and their families will be related to more general theoretical and political themes. Many of the issues informing haemoglobinopathies can only be understood in relation to wider concerns such as family obligation, ethnicity, chronic illness and disability (Ahmad and Atkin 1996b). This enhances current debates about sickle cell and thalassaemia by providing a broad framework to make sense of the experience of living with a chronic illness. As we argued in Chapter 1, previous work on sickle cell and thalassaemia often fails to provide a contexualized account and as a consequence ignores many important insights that could help improve our understanding of haemoglobinopathies. Such an approach also establishes possible political alliances by identifying potential similarities with other individuals and groups who also experience disadvantage (Penna and O'Brien 1996).

This chapter begins by sketching out these broader themes. These themes will then inform our specific discussion about the experience of living with a sickle cell or thalassaemia disorder. The emerging narrative, however, is not intended as a straightforward description of the literature but more an example of 'thick description', which presents the experience of individuals and their families as multilayered, dynamic and context specific (Geetz 1983). There is no 'one' experience of haemoglobinopathies that can be easily related. Social reality is far more complex than this. Consequently, the experience of individuals and their families is specifically illustrated by discussing discrete, although interrelated examples – such as the impact of haemoglobinopathies on affected individuals, family relationships and coping – within the broader social context. The emerging and interwoven narratives offer an insight into how SCD and thalassaemia affect the lives of individuals and their families and perhaps provide a better reflection of their experience than simply listing the various difficulties presented by the condition. The next chapter will then carry these ideas forward and discuss the role and organization of health and social care for affected individuals and their families.

Disability, chronic illness and the family

Disability and chronic illness

Living with a haemoglobinopathy has similarities with other forms of disability and chronic illness (Thompson 1994a). There is, however, a theoretical and political tension between 'chronic illness' and 'disability' (Oliver 1996). Disability is often defined in terms of physical or mental impairment, whereas chronic illness is characterized as a steady state with periods of severe ill health. In practice, however, such a distinction is often difficult to maintain (Ahmad 2000). SCDs and thalassaemia, for example, can be seen as a chronic illness with disabling consequences, some of which we described in the previous chapter. Exploring this offers a useful starting point in making sense of the politics of sickle cell and thalassaemia as well as an individual's specific illness experience.

Haemoglobinopathies share various features thought to be characteristic of a chronic illness. These include the long-standing nature of the two conditions, uncertainty, clinical consequences which result in a 'steady state' and occasional 'crisis', and the need for regular and lifelong medical surveillance and intervention to limit the consequences of the conditions (see Locker 1997). Not surprisingly, chronic illness impacts on daily living, social relationships and self-identity (Locker 1997), reducing a person's capacity to pursue activities regarded as normal for their age and gender (see Davis and Wasserman 1992). To this extent, illness is a stressor (Hurtig and White 1986) and the mainstream literature on chronic illness provides an analytical framework, which can make further sense of an individual's experience. When people speak about their illness it becomes evident that their experiences of illness are woven into biographies (Williams 1984), reflecting their experience of life (Cowen et al. 1984). This 'illness narrative' (Kleinman 1988) gives voice to people's attempts to deal with their life situation and the problems of identity that chronic illness may bring (Hyden 1997). Narratives, in effect represent and reflect this experience, as well as making sense of the relationship between the person's body, self and illness (Bury 1991). Further, they reflect the struggle to lead valued lives and maintain a definition of self that is positive and worthwhile (Locker 1997).

Despite the merits of relating haemoglobinopathies to the broader chronic illness literature, the 'handicaps' associated with the illnesses suggest there is also value in conceptualizing haemoglobinopathies as a disability within the context ascribed by the 'disability movement' (Oliver 1996).[1] Many of the problems faced by individuals and their families are socially constructed and are appropriately discussed within the broader context of discrimination and disadvantage faced by disabled people. Following this, several black disabled activists regard haemoglobinopathies as a disability and suggest more established links with mainstream disabled organizations (Begum 1994; Stuart 1996).

The wider society, for instance, often views haemoglobinopathies as a personal tragedy and ignores the ways in which the disadvantages faced by those with the illness are socially determined (see Finkelstein 1993). As part of this, people with a haemoglobinopathy find their experience subordinated to a discourse that defines their problems as purely medical. This is a common form of disadvantage facing disabled people and an important consideration in mobilization (Oliver 1996). The dominance of medical discourse often estranges an individual from their own body and reifies the illness experience. This means that the individual can find themselves excluded from decisions taken about their lives (Corker and French 1998) and their views are ignored in discussion about how their illness is treated or managed (Atkin 1991).

Disabilist discourses are also evident in other ways. As part of living with their illness, individuals have to deal with the response of the formal organizations in the wider society (Shakespeare 1999). People with SCD and thalassaemia may find that educational institutions cannot accommodate the consequences of their condition (Vlachou 1997). They may also find themselves excluded from certain types of social activity and employment, as well as experience discrimination in their dealings with financial agencies such as mortgage and insurance companies, because of the inflexible attitudes of the wider society (Black and Laws 1986; Atkin and Ahmad 2000a, 2000b). This becomes the basis of social exclusion, and another important mobilizing force for disabled people (Oliver 1996; Shakespeare 1999).

It is worthwhile to consider the example of employment in more detail as exclusion from the labour market is at the heart of disabled politics (Lunt and Thornton 1997). In western societies, employment plays an important role in defining a person's identity and offers material rewards (Roulstone 1998). To this extent, work is an important component of adult life and difficulties in gaining employment are frequently associated with indicators of distress in other areas of life (Midence and Elander 1994). Financial pressures, for instance, can precipitate emotional and psychological problems. A stimulating and fulfilling working life, on the other hand, can help maintain self-confidence and self-image as well as compensate for disruptions in other areas of life (Lunt and Thornton 1997). Disabled people, however, find it difficult to gain fulfilling and financially rewarding employment because employers' views reflect the wider society's ignorance, inflexibility and inability to accommodate difference (Oliver 1996). Those with haemoglobinopathies face these disadvantages and discrimination. Their problems are further compounded by the more general discrimination faced by minority ethnic groups when they look for work (Craig and Rai 1996).

The need for occasional absences is one of the main difficulties, faced by those with a haemoglobinopathy, in achieving a stable employment record (Franklin and Atkin 1986). This remains a major worry for those with a SCD or thalassaemia. It is important, however, that potential restrictions in access to employment are kept to a minimum, as Whitten and Fischoff (1974: 687) explain:

> The disease also imposes a sense of insecurity, for adults are quite aware that sickle cell anaemia may result in disqualification for a job or a dismissal after hiring. Because of the role of work and self-sufficiency in the development of the individual's social identity, any factor that works against the acquisition and retention of a meaningful job has the potential for undermining or destroying a previously good psychosocial adjustment.

This is equally true for those with thalassaemia (Atkin and Ahmad 2000c). Moreover, problems with work generally translate into problems with money (Midence and Elander 1994) and such financial constraints tend to work against chronically ill and disabled people more than 'healthy' individuals (Hirst and Baldwin 1994). Many people with haemoglobinopathies, for instance, live on low incomes, yet may have to meet additional outgoings, because of the very consequences that limit their income (Black and Laws 1986). They may also suffer:

> when for financial reasons they are not able to keep a car, keep their central heating on for long periods of the year, or go on holiday, or when they live in damp or draughty accommodation, climb flights of stairs, or contend with disputes about registration as citizens and perhaps face deportation.
>
> (Midence and Elander 1994: 100–1)

Consequently, a more sensitive employment policy for those with haemoglobinopathies could make the difference between a successful coping strategy and one characterized by dependence, poor self-image and feelings of helplessness (Midence and Elander 1994). This is also a common argument employed by people with other forms of disability, who cite evidence that suggests disabled people are less likely to be afforded the same rights as able-bodied workers in accessing jobs, equal employment rights and equal access to the workplace (Roulstone 1998).

The role of active agency and family caregiving

Current writings on disability and chronic illness, both in their different ways, present individuals as active agents, exercising control over their lives. As we have seen, the disability movement constructs this active agency within a more political framework (Oliver 1996), whereas those writing on chronic illness emphasize the role of the individual making sense of their illness within a social context (Conrad and Bury 1997). Both approaches, however, give primacy to the individual and their experience and no doubt this proves valuable when discussing haemoglobinopathies. This is especially evident when discussing children, whose voices are rarely heard in discussion about disability or chronic illness (Morris 1998) or in debates about haemoglobinopathies (Bailey-Holgate 1996; Anie *et al.* 2000; Atkin and Ahmad 2000b, 2000c). A 9-year-old girl with a haemoglobinopathy, who had not been invited to a workshop for young adults with SCD and thalassaemia but managed to attend, commented:

> This is my condition. I am the one who has to live with it. I cannot see why adults should decide what I need to know about it and when to tell me. I have feelings too. All I want is to have my questions answered when I ask, to have my parents listen to how I feel so that I do not bottle up and hide my feelings; to be told everything about my condition. I will say if I do not understand.
>
> (Bailey-Holgate 1996: 500)

There is, however, a tension in asserting individual rights of disabled and chronically ill people and the primacy of their experience. The increasingly powerful critique of the disability movement, despite its obvious merits in asserting the rights of disabled people, tends to be dismissive of family care by arguing that policy should not endorse dependence on family caregivers but underwrite the independence of the disabled person (Oliver 1996). This approach is perhaps understandable, given that the state often advocates family care at the expense of considering how best to achieve optimal independence for the disabled person and their family (Twigg and Atkin 1994). Disabled people and their carers, however, both have to face the consequences of this policy and experience disadvantages that prevent them from enjoying the same opportunities as most other people. This would make disabled people and their carers natural allies, rather than discrete groups competing against each other for limited resources (Ahmad 2000). For their part, carers' groups are perhaps as guilty in maintaining this opposition as disabled organizations, by implicitly presenting disabled people as a 'burden'.

Simplistic constructions of the opposition between carers and disabled people have been challenged (Parker 1993; Ahmad 2000). At its most straightforward, the provision of support to replace family care, for example, may run counter to what the disabled person wants. Disabled people, for example, rarely choose to reject the care of close family, especially if they share the same household. This argument, although applying generally, may have particular implications for minority ethnic disabled people and their families (Ahmad 1996a). Members of disability movement have been slow to consider ethnicity and many of their arguments about independent living may not have the same meaning for minority ethnic groups (Ahmad 2000). To this extent, young Asian and African-Caribbean people in the UK construct their identities in the context of both their ethnic and religious culture as well as the broader British culture (see Modood *et al.* 1994).

Research on the experience of young people with a haemoglobinopathy confirms this approach to identity construction. As they grow older, young people are keen to assume what they regard as adult roles, in the British context, by asserting their independence and own identity (Brannen *et al.* 1994; Frydenberg 1997). To this extent, South Asian and African-Caribbean young people with a haemoglobinopathy do feel they have to develop and sustain an identity separate from their parents and exercise some control over their own lives (Atkin and Ahmad 2000b, 2000c). Differences, however, also occur. Comparing the narratives of African-Caribbean respondents (Atkin and Ahmad 2000b) as well as the more general literature on young people (Brannen *et al.* 1994) with South Asian young people, suggests concerns about leaving home and establishing an independent existence assumed less importance for South Asian young people (Atkin and Ahmad 2000b). Minority ethnic young people may be more likely to emphasize self-sufficiency within the family than white young people (Brannen *et al.* 1994).

This offers a more general reminder that arguments about 'independence' do not reflect adequately how many people experience disability or chronic illness. Consequently it is not possible to focus on the needs of the individual in isolation from the family context (Twigg and Atkin 1994), irrespective of ethnic origin (Atkin and Rollings 1996). Not only is the care of an individual negotiated within the context of obligations and reciprocities (Finch and Mason 1993), but people themselves rarely take decisions about their health and lifestyles independently of their families (Graham 1984). More specifically, the influence of family members on each other and their different roles within their family have long been recognized as affecting the functioning of the whole family (Minuchin 1974). This does not deny the individual's personal perspective nor does it negate their right to independent living. Rather it recognizes the role of family in shaping the experience of the individual (Midence *et al.* 1996) and the important role of the family in supporting disabled and chronically ill people (Twigg and Atkin 1994).

Consequently, both the affected individual and their family have to cope with disability and chronic illness. This does not suggest a unified experience, as the implications of the condition can be very different for those who have it and those who provide support. Nonetheless, each has their own distinct narrative that contributes to the politics of sickle cell and thalassaemia. The relevance of this can be seen throughout the chapter.

Coping with a chronic illness

Neither individuals nor their families are passive victims of circumstance but engage with their illness, employing social, cultural and material resources to overcome the difficulties they face (Beresford 1996b). That people with a chronic illness and their families face considerable physical, emotional and financial stress is well supported (Baldwin and Carlisle 1994) and is documented throughout this book. Nonetheless there is an increasing interest in how individuals and families cope, using varying strategies and with varying degrees of success, with chronic illness rather than simply describing the 'burdens' of their life. Consequently, there is considerable emphasis on the cognitive and behavioural strategies that people use to deal with the demands of everyday life (Eiser 1994). Individuals and their families are highly creative – using various resources and strategies – in managing and overcoming difficulties (Frydenberg 1997).

The experience of living with a haemoglobinopathy, therefore, seems more appropriately discussed in the context of coping (Ahmad and Atkin 1996b). This emphasizes the materials, resources and strategies – at personal, social and professional levels – which are found helpful in providing optimum care in a way that is most beneficial to the individual as well as other family members (Beresford 1994). Such an approach is especially important in understanding how services can best support people, by underwriting the individuals' and their families' existing strengths (Ahmad and Atkin 1996b). On the other hand, an emphasis on coping should not be used as an excuse to ignore the difficulties faced by young people and parents. To this extent, coping should not be perceived as an individual achievement or failing (Atkin and Ahmad 2000a). Nor should coping be considered in isolation of social or service support, particularly since a clear source of stress within families frequently arose from having to manage the demands of caring with insufficient support from services (Sloper and Turner 1993a). The next chapter discusses this further.

Despite these provisos, an emphasis on coping and active agency enables us to place an individual's experience within a broader social context and reminds us that having a haemoglobinopathy is only one aspect of their identity. Individuals and their families, for example, have the same aspirations and worries as the general population (Anionwu 1993). Their illness does not excuse them from conforming to societal roles, norms and expectations (Scambler 1996). People with SCD and thalassaemia have to find employment, establish and maintain social networks, assume the roles of spouses, parents, siblings and children. Having a chronic illness may complicate this process (Bury 1991) but it does not fundamentally alter it (Williams 1984). Adopting such an approach allows us to move beyond simplistic accounts that associate chronic illness with 'burden' (Beresford 1994). Disabled or chronically ill individuals and their families are sometimes seen as different and in some instances, even dysfunctional (Moore *et al.* 1997) or pathological (Atkin 1991). Individuals and their families are not seen as people fulfilling family obligations, but as people whose lives were severely disrupted by disability (Parker 1993). This, however, is not how individuals or families experience their illness (Atkin *et al.* 1998a). Although chronic illness can be seen as a stressor, the impact on self-image is neither inevitable, universal nor consistent (Zani *et al.* 1995). Individuals and their families, for example, strive to limit the impact of the illness on their lives (Twigg and Atkin 1994; Locker 1997) and disability or chronic illness does not necessarily have to dominate all aspects of an individual's life (Morris 1991). The great majority of families with a disabled person experience the same emotions, bonds, joys and pleasures of family life as families with a non-disabled member, as well as the same pains, conflicts and disappointments (Beresford *et al.* 1996). This is why, for example, parents of disabled children often say they see their *child* first and the *disability* second (Beresford 1994).

The experience of young people growing up with chronic illness can illustrate this further. Chronic illness, although disruptive, is only one of the many competing concerns they face (Atkin and Ahmad 2000b, 2000c). All young people have to cope with the new experiences and responsibilities of growing up (Dornbusch *et al.* 1991) as well as developing more complex emotional relationships and social interactions (Sawyer *et al.* 1995). This is irrespective of whether the child has a chronic illness or not. During this process the young people assume different social roles and expectations, establish their own identity and assert their growing sense of independence (Noller and Callan 1991). Emotional difficulties emerge in response to the real problems such as negotiating with parents, establishing peer relationships, coping with school, and making decisions about future ambitions (Brannen *et al.* 1994; Anie *et al.* 2000). Chronic illness certainly complicates this, but cannot be divorced from the general experience of growing up (Ebata and Moss 1991). This is why young people with a haemoglobinopathy express similar concerns and anxieties as well as aspirations to young people who do not have a chronic illness (Atkin and Ahmad 2000c). Such tensions continue into adulthood as an individual considers establishing intimate relationships and the possibility of marriage, starting a family, running a household, finding employment and pursuing a career (Midence and Elander 1994). We will return to this when we discuss family relationships.

Ethnicity and disadvantage

Up to now we have discussed the experience of SCD and thalassaemia within the general context of chronic illness and disability. One of the important features of haemoglobinopathies in the UK, as we have seen, is that they occur almost exclusively among minority ethnic groups and this necessarily mediates the illness experience (Bradby 1996; Dyson 1998). First, the general disadvantages and inequalities facing minority ethnic groups mean that the impact of chronic illness may be greater. Financial restrictions and poor housing, for example, are potential contributory factors to poor coping for those with a chronic illness (Beresford 1994). Yet inequalities in income, employment and housing are well documented among minority ethnic groups (Skellington 1992; Owen 1994). Though far from homogenous, income levels of South Asian and African-Caribbean people are lower than the UK average and their unemployment rates are about twice those in the white population (Craig and Rai 1996; Modood *et al.* 1997). Further, 28 per cent of white households have incomes below half the national average; this compares to 84 per cent of Bangladeshi families, 82 per cent of Pakistani families, 45 per cent of Indian families and 41 per cent of African-Caribbean families (Modood *et al.* 1997). Minority ethnic families are also less likely to receive their full social security entitlement (Law 1996) and this, as we shall see in the next chapter, is a particular issue in haemoglobinopathies. Further, formal service support – another important feature of successful coping – is likely to be inaccessible and less appropriate for minority ethnic communities (Ahmad and Atkin 1996b). As we have seen, for instance, the neglect of haemoglobinopathies is often attributed to its association with minority ethnic groups and the inability of health and social care agencies to meet the needs of people from these groups. The next chapter on service delivery explores these issues in greater detail.

Second, cultural identity is an important mediator of the experience of chronic illness. Conceptions of health and illness involve symbolic forms, beliefs and values and there are cultural differences in both ideas and behaviour relating to health and illness (Currer 1986; Helman 2000). A focus on identity and culture also reminds us that we cannot ascribe the same imperatives to all ethnic groups. Ideas about childhood, autonomy and independence, as we have seen, are social and cultural constructions, reflecting different accounts of family obligation and reciprocities across ethnic groups (see also Ahmad 1996b, 2000; Katbamna *et al.* 2000). To add to the complexity these ideas are also open to different interpretations across people and across time, and are structured by social cleavages, previous experience, relationships, resources and priorities (Ahmad 1996b). Social class, gender relations and the process of social change are also important factors in influencing norms and behaviour. In the same way, the reproduction of culture, for example, does not constitute implanting the norms, behaviours and aspirations of one generation to the next (Ahmad 1996b). Reproduction is dynamic, involving negotiation and engagement. It encompasses conflicting values within the family, influences of the wider society, personal agendas of various actors, the role of the economy, legal frameworks and the impact of and resistance to a racialized external world (Anthias 1992).

Until recently, however, cultural accounts were often dismissed as a surrogate form of racism because of the way they simplified and pathologized the experience of minority ethnic people. (The next chapter discusses the influences of such approaches and highlights their negative impact on the lives of minority ethnic people.) Crude multiculturalism stripped minority ethnic cultures of their dynamism, vitality, flexibility and variability and offered these as rigid determinants of individual and group desires and behaviours (Centre for Contemporary Cultural Studies 1982). There is, however, a growing realization that the conceptualization of culture was the problem rather than culture per se (Ballard 1989). For example, explaining adversity as relating to God's will has sometimes been confused with an abdication of responsibility and despondency among minority ethnic groups (Kelleher and Hillier 1996) rather than a valuable coping resource (Atkin and Ahmad 2000c). Empirical accounts, for example, make clear that illness is not passively accepted and that people assume responsibility for their own health (Currer 1986; Hillier and Rahman 1996; Kelleher and Islam 1996; Lambert and Sevak 1996).

More generally, a re-evaluation of culture enables a more considered explanation of how people perceive and manage their illness (Smaje 1995). The grounded experiences and active agency of the subject is thus restored by focusing on the meanings and interpretations through which people make sense of their world (Chamba *et al.* 1998). As such, cultural background informs people's norms and actions, as they make sense of what is happening around them (Ahmad 1995, 1996a; for a more general discussion see Finch and Mason 1993). Cultural sensitivity, therefore, needs to be an important feature of our discussion about haemoglobinopathies. We will return to this topic.

Living with a haemoglobinopathy

After setting out the general concerns and themes informing debates about disability and chronic illness, we now turn our specific attention to haemoglobinopathies. The subsequent discussion builds on the general concerns and themes outlined above to provide an insight into how individuals and their families make sense of living with SCD or thalassaemia. As with other chronic illnesses, SCD and thalassaemia impose lifelong restrictions to which the individual must learn to adapt. For example, individuals must acquire skills and knowledge relevant to their condition and its control if they are to take responsibility for the management of their condition and avoid serious complications (Eiser 1994; Hill 1994). They must also come to terms emotionally with the condition and any limitations it imposes (Barbarin *et al.* 1994; Wjst *et al.* 1996). Feelings of isolation, dependence, fear of illness, withdrawal from normal relationships with peers and family as well as poor self-image, depression and preoccupation with death are common themes in the haemoglobinopathy literature (Midence and Elander 1994).

In early childhood, relationships with family and peers may be disrupted by episodes of chronic sickness (Hanson *et al.* 1989; Hurtig 1994). In later childhood, a chronic illness may hamper progress in education and the achievement of independence from the family (Conyard *et al.* 1980; Midence 1994). The emotional concerns of the teenage years may be compounded by delayed growth, worries about sexual development, and more generally, aspirations of adult life may have to be revised in the light of the limitations imposed by the condition (Hurtig and White 1986; Darr 1990). The teenage years are also a time when young people with chronic or disabling conditions become aware of their difference and the difficulties they may face (Telfair 1994). Non-use of the infusion pump is particularly common among teenagers with thalassaemia, as they strive to be 'normal', adopt lifestyles that are consistent with their own wishes and identities and are valued by their peers, and take greater personal control of their own care (Ratip and Modell 1996; Atkin and Ahmad 2000c). More generally children, as they reach their teens, may reject what they regard as other people's (including parents' and professionals') definitions of what is in their interests (Blum 1992; Hill 1994; Phelps and Jarvis 1994). They also have to face the dilemma of how to reconcile a growing wish for independence with the threat of increased illness-related dependence (Sinnema 1992).

This dilemma is carried through into adult life and finds expression in newfound responsibilities and aspirations (Midence and Elander 1994). Adults with SCD, for example, report that their illness affects their social activities and undermines their ability to maintain social networks (Black and Laws 1986). Their illness also means that many of the social and leisure activities, taken for granted by those without a haemoglobinopathy, must be treated with caution. These include physical exertion, getting wet or chilled, swimming, high altitude and even heavy meals (Midence and Elander 1994). Adults may also suffer socially because of their fear of stigmatization (Broome and Monroe 1979; Darr 1990; Anionwu 1993). People, for example, describe much prejudice and ignorance when they tell others they have a haemoglobin disorder (Anionwu 1993). Popular myths include an association with HIV and AIDS and a fear that their illness is contagious. Concerns about stigma can be carried over into attempts to establish significant and meaningful relationships. A particular worry among those with a haemoglobinopathy, for instance, is whether partners would be able to cope with their illness (Anionwu 1993: Midence and Elander 1994; Atkin and Ahmad 2000b). There are then more general difficulties associated with maintaining a household, starting a family, assuming parental responsibilities and earning a living (Midence and Elander 1994; Ahmad and Atkin 1996b). All can be disrupted by the consequences of either SCD or thalassaemia.

More generally – and regardless of age – quality of life can be affected by anxieties about the future (Midence and Elander 1994), which introduces another fundamental aspect of haemoglobinopathies: *uncertainty* (Locker 1997). The management of uncertainty becomes a major aspect of families' experience, especially in SCD (Midence 1994). As we have seen, the clinical consequences of haemoglobinopathies are *probable* rather than *definite*; SCD, in particular, is variable and episodic. Health professionals cannot say with any degree of certainty what the consequences of SCD or thalassaemia will be. Individuals and their families therefore have to constantly juggle the hope of relief and remission against the apprehension of disease progression (Headings 1976). We will return to this when we discuss the vulnerability of coping strategies.

The relationship between haemoglobinopathies and psychological problems, however, is far from straightforward (Fowler *et al.* 1986; Swift *et al.* 1989; Midence *et al.* 1996). Several studies have failed to find differences in psychological coping between children with haemoglobinopathies and children with no chronic illness (Kumar *et al.* 1976; Lemanek *et al.* 1986; Vullo *et al.* 1995; Zani *et al.* 1995; Hilton *et al.* 1997). Differences, when they did occur, could be attributed to social and economic factors, such as poverty and minority status, rather than factors related to the illness (Lemanek *et al.* 1986; Molock and Belgrave 1994). Indeed several studies demonstrate how individuals can have a positive self-image and cope with the condition successfully (Midence and Elander 1994; Zani *et al.* 1995). These seemingly contradictory research findings suggest that some individuals with SCD or thalassaemia may be at risk of developing psychological problems, but others are not (Politis *et al.* 1990; Barbarin *et al.* 1994; Midence 1994), which is consistent with the general literature on chronic illness (Mador and Smith 1989; Wjst *et al.* 1996). The findings also suggest that an individual's response to their illness could change over time and we explore this in more detail below. Although there are times when individuals do get down, most of the time they are able to cope successfully with the limitations imposed by their illness. A more relevant research question, therefore, would be how individuals cope with a chronic illness and what are the threats to their coping strategies (Midence and Elander 1994). This seems a more appropriate way of discussing the illness narrative and we return to this later in the chapter when we explore the coping strategies adopted by affected individuals and their families.

Haemoglobinopathies and family life

As we have seen, an individual's experience is inevitably linked to the experience of other family members. This becomes an important consideration in making sense of haemoglobinopathies. The role of parents is especially important (Sloper and Turner 1993b) and their influence is usually evident throughout an individual's life (Atkin 1992). An individual, for example, not only has to accommodate their own anxieties and concerns but also those of their parents (Midence and Elander 1994). At the same time, having a child with a haemoglobinopathy can have long term consequences for parents (Ahmad and Atkin 1996b) and it is to these we first turn.

Caring for a child with a haemoglobinopathy, although involving less physical tending than many other chronic illnesses and disabilities, still has social and psychological consequences for the parent. These can continue throughout the parent's life and do not end, for example, when the child leaves home. The literature documents a range of emotions experienced by parents. These include guilt, frustration, anxiety, helplessness, loneliness, isolation and resentment (Quine and Pahl 1985; Baldwin and Carlisle 1994). The more specific literature on sickle cell and thalassaemia documents feelings of hopelessness and frustration, especially during diagnosis and over uncertainty about prognosis (Whitten and Fischoff 1974; Anionwu and Beattie 1981; May and Choiseul 1988; Midence and Elander 1994; Atkin et al. 1998b). The genetic nature of SCD and thalassaemia can also mean that parents may feel guilty about having passed the condition on to their child (Anionwu and Jibril 1986; Vullo et al. 1995; Atkin et al. 2000). Interestingly, however, this does not concern those with the condition and they do not usually use the inherited nature of the condition against their parents. Many with the illness, however, do admit there are times when they take out their frustrations on their parents (Atkin and Ahmad 2000b, 2000c) and this is something else parents have to deal with. Again, this appears to be a key feature of growing up with a chronic illness (Geiss et al. 1992), as well as growing up more generally (Brannen et al. 1994).

In both SCD and thalassaemia, parents express more general concerns about the child's future (Telfair et al. 1994) and such worries can become a defining feature of the parents' role (Atkin et al. 2000). All parents, for example, worry about the condition getting worse and the possibility of an early death as well as about the implications of the child's condition for their future social role (Atkin and Ahmad 2000a). Parental worries do not stop when the child reaches adulthood. Poor quality service provision can make the stress of caring worse. Parents, for example, feel they have to fight constantly in order to obtain appropriate care for their child (Atkin et al. 1998a). Indeed, some parents felt that professionals were insensitive or racist. The next chapter explores this perception further.

All parents find caring stressful and demanding, but accept that they have to cope with the situation for the sake of the child (Atkin et al. 2000). To this extent parents emphasize the importance of getting on with daily living – a theme common in other studies on family caregiving (Lewis and Meredith 1988). Most parents, therefore, emphasize the importance of accepting their caring responsibilities and coping with things as they happen (Atkin *et al*. 2000). This, as we shall see, is similar to the coping strategies adopted by those with the illness.

Besides these social and psychological consequences, haemoglobinopathies can also have material consequences for families of affected individuals. This could have implications for family life, as financial restrictions are a potential contributory factor to poor coping in childhood (Midence and Elander 1994). Parents, especially the mother's ability to earn income, can be reduced because of the consequences of their caregiving role (Atkin *et al*. 2000). Mothers, for example, may have to take time off work or only work part time as they care for their child. Fathers may have to take unpaid time off work to accompany their child to hospital or to help out the mother when the child falls ill. Racial inequalities in income and employment often mean the financial impact of care may even be greater for minority ethnic families (see above).

Housing is another important factor in the overall environment of providing care. Poor housing can threaten a child's health, as well as affect the ease with which parents can meet the child's care needs (Beresford 1996a). Damp and draughty housing, lack of appropriate heating and the financial inability to keep the house warm would be significant problems in looking after a child with SCD or thalassaemia (Black and Laws 1986). Certain types of housing (such as high rise flats or accommodation over several floors) can also limit the children's and parents' lives considerably (Ahmad and Atkin 1996a). Again, housing inequalities often exacerbate the problems for minority ethnic families, who are more likely to live in older unmodernized, inner city housing lacking in household amenities such as central heating, washing machines and gardens (Owen 1994; see also above).

The relationship between parent and child
The relationship between a parent and their child offers another important means of making sense of how individuals and their families live with a haemoglobinopathy. Young children seem to describe a close and loving relationship with their parents and to this extent, parents are an important coping resource, enabling the young person to come to terms with his or her illness (Atkin and Ahmad 2000b, 2000c). This support involves both mother and father (Atkin and Ahmad 2000a). Fathers, although less involved than mothers – who tend to assume main responsibility for care – still provide a valuable support role (Atkin *et al*. 2000). This helps counter the myth of the distant or absent father common to accounts of Asian and African-Caribbean family life (Midence and Elander 1994).

Parents and their children, however, can have different views on the consequences of the condition. When asked about the impact of sickle cell disease in the family, children are more likely to indicate negative feelings than parents (Hurtig 1994). Parents, for example, tend to down play the consequences of the condition in their attempt to exercise some control over it (Hill 1994). For their part, children may also hide the consequences of the illness from their parents (Thompson 1994a) and this continues into adulthood (Midence and Elander 1994). This is perhaps unfortunate because the more a parent is able to discuss the condition with their child, the better able the child is to cope with their chronic illness (Clarfin and Barbarin 1991).

More generally, young people are often aware of the consequences of their condition but if their parents have not discussed this with them, they feel unable to bring the topic up (Clarfin and Barbarin 1991). Young people are concerned to protect their parents and not add to their problems. Young people therefore believe they have to cope with the illness alone and are reluctant to ask questions, clarify concerns or share information (Eiser 1994). Interestingly, we know that parents adopt a similar strategy and also seek to protect the child. This means that an uneasy truce emerges, where affected individuals and their parents wish to discuss the illness, but feel unable to do so unless the other mentions it first (Atkin and Ahmad 2000a, 2000b).

As the child gets older they also have to negotiate independence as they make sense of the life transitions associated with growing up. This, as we have seen, is an important part of being a young person and occurs in all families – regardless of whether the child has a chronic illness or not (Frydenberg 1997). General disagreements between parents and young people are frequent during this process, with the young person attempting to assert their own identity and negotiate their autonomy (Dornbusch *et al.* 1991). This is perhaps why the arguments between children with a haemoglobinopathy and their parents are similar to general arguments that occur during childhood (Ahmad and Atkin 1996b). In the same way, young people, as they seek to develop their own life views and identities, may reject their parents' definitions of what is in their interests (Frydenberg 1997). Again, this occurs irrespective of chronic illness and offers another reminder that family life offers more than simply a framework in which to engage with chronic illness.

As we have discussed above, a child with a chronic illness can still take an active part in family life as a son or a daughter or a brother or a sister (Beresford *et al.* 1996). In the same way, what goes on in households between parents and young people concerning rule setting, negotiation and control is no different from what happens between parents and young people with a chronic illness (see Thompson 1994a). Young people with an SCD or thalassaemia, for example, have to negotiate life transitions in the same ways as their peers as they assume responsibility for their lives (Brannen *et al.* 1994). Coping with the emerging expectations and responsibilities of growing up is common among all young people (Jenks 1994) and to this extent young people's illness narratives become negotiated within the context of family relationships as well as the normative expectations of what it is to be a young person (also see above).

Nonetheless, the experience of a chronic illness can make the negotiation of responsibility and autonomy particularly fraught (Midence and Elander 1994). For example, parents may have to supervise a child's medication and ensure they follow various precautions. These can become sites of struggle as a child gets older (Atkin *et al.* 2000) and can cause particular tensions between child and parent (Ratip *et al.* 1995). Non-use of the infusion pump is especially common among adolescents with thalassaemia, as they strive to be 'normal', adopt lifestyles that are consistent with their own wishes and identities and are valued by their peers, and take greater personal control of their own care (Ratip and Modell 1996; Atkin and Ahmad 2000c). Parents said that the most frequent cause of arguments with their teenage offspring was the use of the infusion pump and they never fully trusted their child to comply with their treatment (Atkin *et al.* 2000). Young people – for their part – sometimes feel their parents overreact to their illness (Midence *et al.* 1996). Young people specifically feel there are times when their parents' concerns about the illness allow it to take over their lives. This is why some young people complain that their parents sometimes see the illness rather than them (Atkin and Ahmad 2000b, 2000c). Many parents seem to be aware of this problem but are not sure how to deal with it (Atkin and Ahmad 2000a). These feelings can lead to tensions in the parent–child relationship with young people accusing their parents of being overprotective, a common theme in the literature on childhood disability (Eiser 1990: Davis and Wasserman 1992) as well as the more general literature on growing up (Brannen *et al.* 1994).

Other family relationships
An individual's illness can have a more general impact on family relationships and this can be another important aspect informing the experience of living with a haemoglobinopathy. We know, for example, that the quality of the relationship between mother and family and among other siblings can influence a young person's coping ability (Beresford 1994). Those better able to cope with the condition are more likely to live in close, loving expressive families (Ahmad and Atkin 1996b). The general literature on family caregiving, however, suggests that caring for a disabled child can cause potential tensions within the family, with non-disabled siblings and partners feeling neglected (Quine and Pahl 1985; Parker 1990; Beresford 1994). Mothers particularly worry about neglecting their spouse and other children by concentrating on the needs of the disabled or chronically ill child (Bould 1990). Mothers, especially when the child felt ill, commented on the difficulties of balancing caring for their child with maintaining their more general domestic responsibility and in some cases going out to work (Atkin and Ahmad 2000c). However helpful they felt their spouses and other offspring were, mothers still felt responsible for making sure family life went on. Nonetheless, most mothers seem to fulfil their role well. Following this, strain and conflict between parents and siblings is not inevitable; some experience improvements in the quality of their relationship and

the closeness of the family as a result of having a chronically ill child in the family (Midence and Elander 1994; Beresford 1996b; Tsiantis *et al.* 1996).

SCD and thalassaemia also have a more specific impact on non-affected siblings (Sloper 1996; Darr 1997). Their role in families where a child has a chronic illness or disability is much neglected (Tozer 1996). A Greek study suggested that siblings of thalassaemic children had significantly more psychosocial problems than the control subjects (Labropoulou and Beratis 1995). The same study suggested that siblings of thalassaemic children also scored significantly lower on sports and non-sports activities and on social functioning in terms of the number of friends and number of contacts with them. However, other research would suggest the impact of the condition on siblings was variable, affecting some but not all siblings. Noll *et al.* (1995), for example, found no difference in the social competence of siblings of a child with SCD compared to a control group. This can be perhaps explained by the importance parents of children with a haemoglobinopathy place on treating all siblings the same and of limiting the impact of the illness on family life (Atkin and Ahmad 2000a).

Nonetheless, sharing a household with a disabled or chronically ill member can have an impact on their lives. Siblings, for example, may have to accommodate the disruptions caused by monthly blood transfusions (Darr 1990) or the unpredictability of a painful crisis (Hurtig 1994). As we have seen, parents might also need to give more time to the child with the chronic illness, and consequently other siblings can feel neglected and unsupported (Atkin 1992). At the same time, siblings can also offer valuable support to a disabled or chronically ill child. They can, for example, help their parents with supporting a child with a chronic illness (Glendinning 1985). This may include playing with their sibling, as well as keeping an occasional eye on him or her (Sloper and Turner 1992). Siblings also provide important emotional support, providing someone to talk to other than their parents (Atkin and Ahmad 2000b).

Coping with a haemoglobinopathy

As we have seen, recent research has focused on how individuals and their families cope rather than simply describe the 'burdens' of chronic illness. Following this, the final part of this chapter examines the coping strategies used by individuals as they attempt to make sense of their illness. As we have argued at the beginning of this chapter, this is perhaps a more adequate reflection of how individuals experience chronic illness than cataloguing the many difficulties they face. To begin, however, we will focus on the key factors that facilitate successful coping. These are often wider than individual strategies and illustrate the role of the wider social networks in supporting individuals.

Early diagnosis and appropriate information, the availability of material and social support, and family dynamics are all implicated in successful coping (Darr 1990; Baldwin and Carlisle 1994; Midence and Elander 1994; Kliewer and Lewis 1995). To this extent, psychological coping of individuals with a haemoglobinopathy is similar to that of children with other chronic illnesses (Thompson 1994a). People with SCD and thalassaemia, for example, are reported to hold positive body images if they are living in families that are cohesive, supportive and expressive, and have adequate income to provide the additional necessities of heating, clothing and travel (Midence and Elander 1994). Further, individuals with negative views of their condition are less well able to cope than those who attempt to reduce the effect of the illness on lives by accommodating the positives (Gil *et al.* 1991; Kliewer and Lewis 1995; Midence and Elander 1996).

A clear understanding of the condition on the part of the affected person and their family is also crucial to effective care in the family context as well as appropriate use of health and other services (Baxter *et al.* 1990; Cocking and Athwal 1990; Baldwin and Carlisle 1994) and this is equally true of haemoglobinopathies (Midence and Elander 1994). People with SCD or thalassaemia and their carers often complain about lack of knowledge about the condition, aetiology, prognosis, symptoms and their care and express doubts about the competence, or indeed the willingness, of health professionals to provide such information (Anionwu 1993; Midence and Elander 1994; Atkin *et al.* 1998a).

More generally, appropriate professional support can help reduce stress and facilitate coping by offering practical support with information and financial help, as well as emotional support from professionals themselves or from support groups (Anionwu 1993; Beresford 1994). This is important especially where good family and social networks are not present (Midence and Elander 1994; Kliewer and Lewis 1995). Sloper and Turner (1992) note that contact with services can itself be an important aspect of coping behaviour.

However, negative and unsympathetic responses from professionals, reported in many studies on SCD and thalassaemia, can also be anxiety provoking and exacerbate feelings of isolation, inadequacy and helplessness (Darr 1990; Anionwu 1993). Such experiences also influence families' future use of services (Midence and Elander 1994). Parents of children with SCD, for example, often see service professionals as adding to their problems rather than being a source of support and cite various examples where they have had to deal with insensitive provision (Hill 1994; Atkin *et al.* 1998a). Those with the illness often share this view (Anionwu 1993; Maxwell and Streetly 1998, Maxwell *et al.* 1999). The next chapter explores these issues in more detail.

The response of the wider social network is also implicated in individual coping strategies. As part of living with illness, young people have to deal with the reactions of others (Bury 1991). Supportive social networks and the help of friends can help create a supportive environment from which the individual can gain strength (Beresford 1994). On the other hand, negative responses and the more general possibility of stigma can undermine an individual's coping ability and enforce a negative self-image (Anionwu 1993; also see above). A more general problem facing affected individuals with a haemoglobinopathy and their families is the lack of understanding and knowledge among the general population (Darr 1990; Green and France-Dawson 1997; Lakhani 1999). Other research suggests that some Asian and African-Caribbean people specifically view haemoglobinopathies with a sense of stigma (Anionwu and Beattie 1981; Anionwu 1993) as revealed in a quotation from a respondent in study by France-Dawson (1991):

> Sometimes I ask myself is what we do to make God give us this? He make them take away us lands. He make them take away us freedom. And now he gave us this. Is what we do?

This sense of stigma is reflected in people's disclosure strategies (Atkin and Ahmad 2000c). Most people, for example, are unsure of how others will respond when they are informed about the illness. This explains why most affected individuals do not make an issue of disclosure and will only tell others when they feel it is appropriate to do so. Disclosure, therefore, is often gradual and depends on the level of rapport a person feels they have developed with others. Such an approach also enables affected individuals to maintain a valued self-image by making it clear that their condition is not the only aspect of their identity (see Atkin and Ahmad 2000b, 2000c). Individuals do not want the illness to dominate their life and this, as we shall see, becomes an important coping strategy.

The response of social institutions represents another important aspect of coping with the wider social world. As we have begun to see, many of the disadvantages faced by affected individuals and their families have social causes and are embedded in the institutional practices of society. This explains why haemoglobinopathy services are poor and fail to meet the needs of the individual or his or her family (see Chapters 1 and 6). We shall also see how education services are often unable to accommodate the needs of young people with SCD or thalassaemia (see Chapter 6). Further, as we have seen, employers often do not understand the potential of affected individuals and often discriminate against them (Black and Laws 1986; Franklin and Atkin 1986; Midence and Elander 1994). Affected individuals can also find it difficult to find life insurance or a mortgage (Midence and Elander 1994).

More generally, the response of these social institutions comes to define the social opportunities available to individuals and their families. At its worst, the social disadvantages faced by affected individuals lead to a sense of injustice, reminding people of their difference and contributing to a negative disadvantage (Atkin and Ahmad 2000b, 2000c). It also makes it more difficult to take advantage of the opportunities available in the wider society. Such disadvantage is, of course, related to broader racist discourses, practices and structures, which further add to the discrimination faced by affected individuals and their families (Black and Laws 1986; Ahmad and Atkin 1996b). This is a theme that should now be familiar to us.

Coping with the worries and difficulties associated with haemoglobinopathies

Up to now, we have discussed the broader influences on coping. We now turn to the individual coping strategies employed by affected individuals, as well as their families, as they attempt to come to terms with their illness on a daily basis. Affected individuals do find their illness difficult to cope with but often regard this as a natural response to their condition (Midence 1994). This in itself can be an important coping strategy because the individual feels no different from others with a limiting illness. Nonetheless, having said this, most people say there are times when they ask 'why me?' as they attempt to make sense of their illness (Atkin and Ahmad 2000b, 2000c). This is often, for instance, a child's first response to their difference and one that usually occurs when they reach their teens. They begin to compare themselves with their peers and realize the potential impact of their condition on their attempts to assert independence and maintain their autonomy. Questions, about 'why me?', however, never entirely go away as the child gets older and enters adulthood (Anionwu 1993). Nonetheless, as affected individuals get older, most recognize that asking 'why me?' does not help them come to terms with the long term consequences of their condition and they try to put such questions to the back of their minds. Questioning why the illness happened to them on a regular basis was not regarded as constructive, potentially undermining their self-identity, and ensuring the illness dominated their life (Atkin and Ahmad 2000b, 2000c). Individuals, for example, begin to recognize the importance of working with the illness rather than against it. To this extent, affected individuals develop more successful coping strategies as they get older (Frydenberg 1997), although this is not to say they have learnt to overcome the difficulties associated with their illness. Sadness and frustration can still occur and to this extent individual coping strategies are vulnerable.

For most of the time, people successfully adapt to their illness and cope with the difficulties they face (Ahmad and Atkin 1996a). The importance of this successful coping is increasingly being recognized in literature on chronic illness (Bury 1991; Beresford *et al.* 1996). It seems rare for affected individuals to be constantly overwhelmed by their illness (Midence and Elander 1994; Atkin and Ahmad 2000b, 2000c) and few perceive illness as a *destroyer* on a regular basis (see Herzlich 1973). Most people, although aware that there were times when the illness took over their lives, attempted to ensure their condition did not become a central feature of their lives. This is an important coping strategy when discussing chronic illness (Williams 1984), although it introduces a constant tension in an individual's life: balancing the demands of their illness with the need to ensure it does not become a defining feature of their identity (Locker 1997). This tension also has to be managed by families looking after a child with SCD or thalassaemia (Darr 1997; Atkin *et al.* 2000) and often becomes central to the experience of caregiving (Hill 1994; also see above).

As a way of accommodating this tension, many affected individuals and their families said they tried not to worry about the illness unless something happened and took each day as it came. Such strategies support work suggesting that thalassaemia and SCD do not necessarily adversely affect the psychological development of affected individuals (Politis *et al.* 1990; Hilton *et al.* 1997; also see above). Those with the illness, for instance, try not to dwell on what might have been and say it is important not to become angry and resentful (Black and Laws 1986). As part of this they try to maintain a sense of optimism and play down the negative aspects of the illness. They especially dislike anything that marks out their difference and this allows them to maintain their sense of normalcy and similarity with peers (Atkin and Ahmad 2000b, 2000c).

Attempts to construct normalcy and reduce the impact of the illness on their life, however, can only ever be partially successful. The severity of the condition provides too many reminders of the dangers and limitations affected individuals and their families face. Consequently, individuals and their families are constantly juggling the difficulties associated with their condition and the possibility of relief from the consequences of their illness. To this extent, uncertainty often dominated the experience of individuals and is at the heart of their vulnerability (Hill 1994; also see above).

Attempting to reduce the consequences of living with a chronic illness is part of a dynamic process and explains why a person's ability to cope is constantly shifting; sometimes they can cope with the illness and at other times they cannot. Certainly, there are times when individuals feel at the mercy of the illness and that the world was against them. This is when their sense of difference, anxiety, frustration and powerlessness was especially strong. Most individuals, however, are able to rebuild their coping strategies and reconstruct a distance between themselves and the severity of the illness (Ahmad and Atkin 1996b).

There is often no one cause of a breakdown in an individual's coping strategies. It can be a response to specific life events – often having nothing to do with the illness – that reminds them of their difference and the difficulties they face (Hill 1994). Starting a new school, attempting to find a job, fulfilling family obligations, sustaining close relationships and trying to start a family can underline an individual's sense of difference and cause sadness (Midence and Elander 1994). This offers a further reminder that affected individuals and their families have to cope with a chronic illness within a broader context of maintaining a positive self-image. On other occasions, the severity of the illness can cause the individual to be overwhelmed. To explore this further this chapter will end with a discussion of the impact of pain in SCD and compliance with chelation therapy in thalassaemia. These are often regarded as the defining features of the respective conditions.

Sickle cell disorders and pain

Our discussion of coping has largely focused on the difficulties of living with a chronic illness on a daily basis. The onset of the painful crisis in SCD, however, creates a different set of circumstances with which the affected individual and their family have to cope (Maxwell and Streetly 1998). To this extent, pain requires a practical and emotional response that is quite different from coping with the everyday consequences of SCD. At times, therefore, the painful crisis can be seen as one aspect of the illness, while at other times it *is* the illness.

The possibility of the painful crisis also contributed to the vulnerability of coping strategies and introduced a sense of uncertainty. Individuals and their families had not only to deal with *the consequences of pain* but the *possibility of pain*. Affected individuals' dread of the pain returning, for example, meant they worried about it even when they were well (Midence and Elander 1994). This is also a common theme of parents' accounts (Atkin *et al.* 1998a).

Those with SCD describe the actual pain as the most difficult aspect of their illness (Thompson 1994a, 1994b) and it can evoke a real fear as well as a sense of panic (Atkin and Ahmad 2000b). Obviously, individuals have somehow to cope directly with the pain. Pain, however, assumes a more symbolic and emotional significance, reminding people of their vulnerability (Atkin and Ahmad 2000b). Individuals begin to feel powerless as well as helpless as they are reminded of the severity of their illness and its impact on their self-identity (Maxwell and Streetly 1998). The onset of pain, for example, reintroduces concerns and anxieties about their future, reminding the person of their dependence on others (Anionwu 1993). The affected person is no longer confident that they can cope with SCD. The pain also reminds them of the precarious nature of their existence and the fragility of their claims to 'normalcy' (Atkin and Ahmad 2000b). Not surprisingly, therefore, the onset of a crisis brings on depression as the affected individual becomes overwhelmed by the illness (Midence and Elander 1994).

Parents describe similar feelings (Atkin *et al.* 1998a). They dislike the painful crisis and describe it as the most difficult aspect of looking after someone with a sickle cell disorder (Hill 1994). Not only does the onset of a crisis cause practical disruptions to employment and family life but it also causes parents emotional distress (Atkin and Ahmad 2000b). Parents, for instance, feel powerless, knowing there is nothing they can do to help their child. Young people, for their part, worry about how their parents cope with their pain and this adds another dimension to coming to terms with pain (Atkin and Ahmad 2000b).

The severity of the pain often requires service support, and this offers another reminder about how service delivery is implicated in individual's coping strategies. People's experience of pain control in hospitals, however, is not wholly positive and many report problems in adequate treatment of pain. Particular problems include delays in treatment of pain, as well as ignorance and insensitivity among health professionals. Sharon Edwards, affected by sickle cell anaemia, provided this recollection of her experiences in the casualty department:

> The problem with Casualty is that you arrive in an awful lot of pain, then they call a doctor; (I always tend to call the haematology doctor so that they are standing by when I get there). Then in Casualty – this is no disrespect to Casualty staff – they have to put up a drip first and then they want to ask your history details, which is already on your file and which they already know. It is very difficult to keep still while the doctor puts in a drip and you are in so much pain. To me the most important thing is getting the pain under control and then you can relax and have the drip put in, you can answer questions and you can be examined. But when they want to examine you first, put the drip in and ask all these questions, it is very difficult. You sometimes tend to lash out at them and they think you are being awkward.
>
> (Edwards 1993: 54)

Sharon, who died in November 1992, was a member of the SMAC working party on Sickle Cell and Thalassaemia and this extract was included in the section of their report entitled Pain Control in Sickle Cell Disorder (Department of Health 1993).

Maxwell *et al.* (1999: 1586) describe various strategies of patients frequently admitted to hospital. This included passivity:

> 'Whenever they [doctors and nurses] say anything to me that I don't like I just let it go by . . . Whatever they want to do, they can just do it to me'.
>
> Aggression also emerged and a minority may resort to verbal and occasionally physical aggression, sometimes due to poor treatment of the painful crisis. 'Every time I come to casualty, he [junior doctor] will send me home . . . one day . . . he cancelled my painkiller and said I would have to go home and I said, "Today I'm not going home" . . . So I held him and I punched him.'

These examples represent long-standing problems in the treatment of pain among those with SCD (Black and Laws 1986; Murray and May 1988; Anionwu 1993; Midence 1994; Elander and Midence 1996; Maxwell and Streetly 1998, Maxwell *et al.* 1999) and the next chapter explores possible reasons for this. Nonetheless, an important point to make here is that services often add to what is already a stressful situation for a person with SCD and are often part of the problem rather than the solution.

Use of chelation therapy

Perhaps not surprisingly, young people with thalassaemia often find the regular use of the infusion pump the most difficult and disruptive aspect of their illness (Beratis 1993; Koch *et al.* 1993; Ratip *et al.* 1995). Young people, for instance, specifically say they hate the pump (Atkin and Ahmad 2000c) and more generally, chelation therapy is symbolic of the difficulties of living with thalassaemia in the same way as the painful crisis is central to the experience of those with SCD. Continuous use of the pump, for example, is seen to be restrictive, imposing limitations on the individuals' day-to-day existence (Ahmad and Atkin 1996b). This in turn affects their self-image (Darr 1990; Atkin and Ahmad 2000c).

How individuals and their families respond to chelation therapy goes beyond the actual task of self-injection, the physical discomfort associated with the procedure or knowledge of the importance of chelation to their survival (Atkin and Ahmad 2000c). These influences should not be completely dismissed, particularly since they are often cited by parents as the reasons for non-compliance (Darr 1990; Atkin *et al.* 1998a).

Chelation therapy also has an emotional significance that comes to symbolize the difficulties of living with thalassaemia, especially for those with the illness. This contributes to non-use as much as practical difficulties (Atkin and Ahmad 2000c). Medical regimens, such as chelation therapy, often mark out an individual's difference and to this extent rejection of compliance can be seen as an attempt to secure normalcy and expressing choice within the broader context of maintaining a valued self-image (Johnson 1988). Unlike parents, not understanding the value of chelation therapy is rarely the issue among those with the illness. Those with thalassaemia usually know the importance of chelation therapy to their well-being, although this is not to say that individuals are deliberately putting themselves at risk. Their response is not as straightforward as this. Individuals with thalassaemia are constantly trying to balance the value of the chelation therapy to their well-being, while at the same time coming to terms with the emotional difficulties caused by its use. This is part of the balancing process noted during our discussion of coping. People with other chronic illnesses seem to face a similar dilemma about medical regimens (Stark *et al.* 1987).

This balancing process is dynamic and explains why their response to chelation therapy is constantly shifting. Usage, although particularly poor among the 13–16 age group for reasons outlined above, still remains varied between individuals and with the same individual over time. There are times when they comply well and others when use is poor. This balance is further influenced by the individual's coping strategies. As we have seen, most coping strategies are generally vulnerable and there are occasions when young people are overwhelmed by the difficulties they face. Not surprisingly, their response to chelation therapy reflects this. The greater the individual's sense of being overwhelmed, the more likely they are to reject chelation therapy (Atkin and Ahmad 2000c).

Conclusion

This chapter outlined the experience of living with a haemoglobinopathy by presenting an 'illness narrative', reflecting the accounts of affected individuals and their families within the broader social, economic and political context. Throughout this chapter, individuals and their families are presented as active agents struggling against disadvantage and discrimination as well as balancing other competing social roles – such as employees, family members and friends – with living with a chronic illness. Empowerment must begin from this premise.

Individuals and their families are highly creative – using various resources and strategies in managing and overcoming the difficulties associated with their illness. Health and social care agencies need to recognize this and help underwrite these strengths by offering support that enables the individual and their families to better accommodate their illness. A better understanding of the problems and difficulties those with the illness and their families face provides an agenda for developing appropriate service support.

At the same time, many of the problems encountered by individuals and their families are a consequence of how the illness is socially perceived. They experience discrimination and disadvantage because of society's inability to accommodate individuals who are 'different'. This disadvantage is informed by racist discourses, which further undermines the position of those with haemoglobinopathies and their families. Strategies are, therefore, required to improve general understanding of SCD and thalassaemia and ensure that social institutions do not discriminate against people with disabilities and chronic illness nor those from minority ethnic groups. Discrimination denies individuals the social opportunities to realize their full potential. Such struggles suggest possible alliances with disability organizations as well as organizations representing specific chronic illness. More generally, racism reminds them that those with haemoglobinopathies are caught up with the broader struggle of minority ethnic groups. The next chapter emphasizes this further by examining the provision of health and social care.

Note

1 The International Classification of Impairments, Disabilities and Handicaps (ICIDH) distinguishes between impairment, disability and handicap (Wood 1980). Impairment is any loss or abnormalcy of psychological, physiological or anatomical structure or function. Disability is a restriction or lack of ability to perform an activity in a manner considered normal for a human being. Handicap is a disadvantage resulting from an impairment or disability that limits or prevents the fulfilment of a role that is normal for that individual. Despite being censured by organizations of disabled people for its uncritical impositions of norms (Oliver 1996) the ICIDH has proved influential in making sense of illness and forms of physical incapacity.

6

Health and social care provision

A user-centred health service would recognise that when people have health problems they do not just have clinical needs, but emotional, psychological, social and financial needs.

(Hogg 1999: 4)

This chapter reviews the literature on the health and social support available to individuals and families with a haemoglobinopathy. In doing so, it identifies specific shortfalls in current provision, many of which are a consequence of failing to understand the narratives of individuals and their families, outlined in the previous chapters. As we have argued throughout the book, rectifying these shortfalls becomes an important focus for strategy and struggle, suggesting a possible agenda for community action as well as state intervention. Many of the themes informing flaws in existing provision will now be familiar to us from our discussion of screening and counselling provision in Chapter 4. Problems revisited in this chapter include poor quality care, inadequate information, insensitivity to the individuals' and families' worries, inappropriate provision, and failure to meet people's needs (Darr 1990; Anionwu 1993; Midence and Elander 1994; Atkin *et al.* 1998b).

At the same time, individuals' high regard for specialist workers and some other health professionals reminds us that services can be sensitive. Examples of good practice do exist and it is important that these influence current provision, providing models for empowerment (Anionwu 1996b; Atkin and Ahmad 2000a). Good practice, as we have argued in previous chapters, not only benefits those with haemoglobinopathies but minority ethnic people and other users in general (McNaught 1987). We would argue that a service that can respond to the needs of the most marginalized sections of society is by definition a good service, better able to cater to all its users. This further illustrates how haemoglobinopathy provision is caught up in the general struggle for more equitable provision faced by minority ethnic groups. To reflect this, the chapter begins by outlining the general difficulties faced by minority ethnic groups in gaining access to appropriate service delivery. It will then specifically focus on haemoglobinopathy provision.

Racism and welfare provision

Debates on health and social care have begun to recognize the particular care needs of Britain's minority ethnic populations. This has been described 'as something of a breakthrough' (Walker and Ahmad 1994), particularly since it occurs against a backdrop of inaccessible and inappropriate service provision (Atkin and Rollings 1993). Conceptually, *institutional racism* emerges as fundamental in explaining the general difficulties faced by minority ethnic families in having their health and social care needs recognized and met by statutory agencies (Ahmad and Atkin 1996a). This, as the opening chapter illustrated, has particular consequences for haemoglobinopathies, especially since their association with minority ethnic groups contributes to their continued neglect.

Institutional racism refers to the policies and practices of an institution leading to racially discriminatory processes or outcomes for users of minority ethnic communities irrespective of the motives of individual employees in the institution (Cashmore and Troyna 1990). Following this, the Macpherson Report (1999: 28) inquiring into the death of Stephen Lawrence defined institutional racism as

> The collective failure of an organisation to provide an appropriate and professional service to people because of their colour, culture, or ethnic origin. It can be seen or detected in processes, attitudes and behaviour which amount to discrimination through unwitting prejudice, ignorance, thoughtlessness and racist stereotyping which disadvantage minority ethnic people.

More specifically, institutional racism has been described as 'camouflaged racism' (Glasgow 1980), meaning it is not open or particularly visible, and is embedded in the taken-for-granted assumptions informing organizational practices.

To this extent, the inability of welfare services to recognize the structural barriers to provision facing minority ethnic people represents a fundamental form of institutional racism. This is manifest in assumptions such as *same service to all*, irrespective of needs, equates with *equal service to all*. Consequently, services are organized according to a 'white norm' and do not recognize difference and diversity, assuming their policies, procedures and practices are equally appropriate for everyone (Atkin and Rollings 1993; Blakemore and Boneham 1995; ALG 2000). Straightforward examples include the inability of health and social services to provide support for people who do not speak English or more specifically the unavailability of vegetarian food or halal meat in day care and domiciliary services. The neglect of haemoglobinopathies is also part of this failure to recognize diversity and difference (Anionwu 1993). More generally, such practices legitimize non-recognition of the needs of minority ethnic communities, disregarding their dietary, linguistic and caring needs (Butt 1994; Bhakta *et al.* 2000; O'Neale 2000).

Another manifestation of institutional racism is the misrepresentation of the needs of ethnic minorities. Health and social services often identify minority ethnic health and social 'problems' as arising from cultural practices (Walker and Ahmad 1994). This results in service organizations blaming minority ethnic communities for the problems they experience. For example, minority ethnic people are frequently characterized as in some way to blame for their own needs because of deviant and unsatisfactory lifestyles (Cameron *et al.* 1989). Indeed there is a history of defining health problems faced by minority ethnic communities in terms of cultural deficits where a shift towards a 'western' lifestyle is offered as the main solution to their problems; examples include the discourses on maternity and child health (Rocherson 1988). Disability, and more generally 'poor birth out-come', among Asian communities has been attributed to consanguineous marriages (Ahmad 1995). As we have seen in Chapter 4, this emerges as a fundamental issue in thalassaemia and health professionals, by emphasizing first-cousin marriage, implicitly blame families for giving birth to a child with thalassaemia (Ahmad *et al.* 2000). We discuss this further below, although it is important to note here that the preoccupation with cultural practices, such as consanguineous marriage, in explaining disability means other important explanations – such as the role of poverty or of services – are rarely mentioned (Atkin 1991). Such an approach also carries an implicit criticism of Asian cultural practices and further creates mistrust between health professionals and their patients (Ahmad *et al.* 2000).

As part of this preoccupation with culture, minority ethnic groups also have to contend with inappropriate generalizations of cultural practices and the use of simplistic explanations to explain their behaviour. Introductory notes on minority ethnic communities, present in most training material for service practitioners, often follow this pattern. One would not, for instance, attempt to summarize a western approach to childrearing practices in one paragraph, yet this is what minority ethnic people are subjected to (Durrant 1989; Jayaratnam 1993). As we have seen in Chapter 4, prenatal diagnosis is sometimes withheld from Muslim families because it is assumed that termination is unacceptable to them. However, like other sections of the population, termination is acceptable to some Muslim families but not to others (Atkin *et al.* 1998b).

Other myths contribute to this failure in recognizing the support needs of South Asian families. A convenient stereotype is that these families virtu-ously 'look after their own' (Atkin and Rollings 1993; Department of Health/ SSI 1998). Health and social care agencies use this as a reason for not planning or providing services for disabled or chronically ill individuals or their families (Walker and Ahmad 1994). The assumption that Asian people live in self-supporting extended family networks is simplistic for a number of reasons (Ahmad 1996a provides a detailed account of these reasons). Household structures, for example, are changing as well as the expectations that inform family obligations. Nonetheless, the assumption that Asian families have the necessary material, emotional and social resources to cope with chronic illness with limited professional support is at best misguided and at worst a racist denial of their support needs (Atkin and Rollings 1996).

Generally, neat cultural packages identifying key characteristics of minority ethnic people do not solve the problems facing community care services and are likely to perpetuate and reinforce cultural stereotypes and myths (Butt 1994; Culley 2000). This, as the previous chapter argues, is not to dismiss the role of cultural identity in informing people's service needs but to challenge accounts that seek to pathologize and simplify cultural practices. This comes to represent an important struggle facing minority ethnic groups (Ballard 1989).

Finally, before leaving this discussion of racism, reference should be made to the potential effect of racist attitudes held by some frontline practitioners. These attitudes can deprive minority ethnic communities of their rights to services, especially since health and social service professionals exercise considerable discretion in their day-to-day work (Lipsky 1980). Racist attitudes on the part of service practitioners have been reported in a number of studies in health and social services (Foster 1988; Cameron *et al.* 1989; Bowler 1993). For example, practitioners working in local authorities often list minority ethnic people as 'high risk' clients, 'uncooperative' and 'difficult to work with' (Cameron *et al.* 1989; Dominelli 1989; Atkin and Rollings 1993). Similarly, evidence suggests that racism within the NHS affects minority ethnic people with common stereotypes, portraying them as 'calling out doctors unnecessarily', 'being trivial complainers', and 'time wasters' (Glendenning and Pearson 1988). As we shall see, these attitudes inform the provision of haemoglobinopathy services and ideas about the 'passivity' of Asian families and 'lower pain thresholds' of African-Caribbean patients deny them the support they need.

Haemoglobinopathy provision

Not surprisingly, haemoglobinopathy services reflect the general problems faced by minority ethnic people in gaining access to appropriate services (Atkin *et al.* 1998a, 1998b). These problems apply equally to young people as well as adults (Anionwu 1996a). Services for SCD and thalassaemia have been described as erratic and lacking in coordination (Prashar *et al.* 1985; Franklin 1988; Streetly *et al.* 1993; Davies *et al.* 1993; Modell *et al.* 2000a). Services that do exist have developed as much in response to community pressure as to rational needs assessment on the part of commissioners or service interests among providers (Atkin *et al.* 1998a). The limited research on service provision documents a variety of problems and these shortfalls in provision mean people with haemoglobinopathies and their families receive inadequate services (Darr 1990; Anionwu 1993; Ahmad and Atkin 1996b; Maxwell and Streetly 1998).

Treatment and support

Inadequate treatment and support is a particular problem facing people with SCD or thalassaemia (Davies *et al.* 1993; Maxwell and Streetly 1998). As we have seen in Chapter 4, early diagnosis, so crucial for adequate care and reducing mortality, remains difficult to obtain. People with SCD or thalassaemia and their carers also express doubts about the ability, or indeed the willingness, of health professionals to provide information so crucial for successful coping (Anionwu 1993; Midence and Elander 1994). Particular problems include difficult to understand information given at what is often regarded by parents as an inappropriate time, an insufficient or rushed explanation, and the lack of opportunity to ask questions about the condition (Darr 1990; Anionwu 1993; Atkin *et al.* 1998b). More generally, professionals who deal with young people are reported to be unsympathetic and to have inadequate knowledge of haemoglobinopathies to provide adequate support (Black and Laws 1986; Shickle and May 1989; Charache and Davies 1991; Anionwu 1993; Midence *et al.* 1996). This lack of knowledge is evident among health care staff as well as schoolteachers, social and youth workers, psychologists and careers advisers. Individuals and their families are especially critical of hospital staff, especially the inexperience and incompetence of junior or non-specialist doctors and nurses (Alleyne and Thomas 1994; Midence and Elander 1994; Ahmad and Atkin 1996b; Maxwell *et al.* 1999).

Nor are these the concerns of 'over-protective parents' and 'over-sensitive individuals' as health professionals and their managers often confirm the difficulties (Atkin *et al.* 1998b). Health professionals agree that some frontline staff know little about haemoglobinopathies and are often insensitive to the needs of individuals and their families (Midence and Elander 1996; Dyson 1997; Atkin *et al.* 1998b; Maxwell and Streetly 1998). Young people and their families, for example, criticize the arrogance of hospital staff who think they know more than the young person about their condition, when they obviously do not (Atkin and Ahmad 2000b). Adults, for their part, are never convinced they are getting the optimal care because of the ignorance of frontline staff (Anionwu 1993; Maxwell and Streetly 1998). These problems create an element of distrust among individuals and their families and a reluctance to use service provision. Many health professionals are felt not to care (Atkin and Ahmad 2000a). It also means that affected individuals and their families feel they have to inappropriately struggle for adequate provision and recognition of their needs (Anionwu 1993). Parents, for example, often describe these battles as the most difficult aspect of caring (Atkin *et al.* 1998a). This is perhaps why individuals and their families emphasize the importance of being assertive and getting to know how the service system works. This, in turn, however, can add to stresses of coping with a chronic illness as well as undermine existing coping strategies.

Individuals' and families' relationship to service provision is also characterized by examples of individual racism (Anionwu 1993). Adults, young people and their families all believe that certain nurses treat them differently from white patients and their families (Darr 1997; Maxwell and Streetly 1998; Atkin and Ahmad 2000b). Individuals with the illness, for example, feel that some health professionals look down on them because of their ethnic identity and make negative judgements about their lifestyles (Black and Laws 1986). Parents cite similar examples and feel their children are often neglected because of their ethnic origin (Atkin and Ahmad 2000a). More generally, affected individuals and their families agree that haemoglobinopathies would receive greater attention if they affected 'white people' (Anionwu 1993). As we have seen, this is noted by many writers on SCD and thalassaemia, who feel that haemoglobinopathies, because they are 'black conditions', are not accorded the same priority as other genetic illness such as cystic fibrosis or haemophilia (see Chapters 1 and 4).

Treating the painful crisis

Patients with SCD, both young people and adults, and their families report specific problems in adequate treatment of pain and believe that most health professionals do not appreciate the severity of painful crisis (Midence 1994; Elander and Midence 1996; Maxwell and Streetly 1998, Maxwell *et al.* 1999 and also see the previous chapter). Anionwu (1993), for example, documents how service providers feel that affected individuals and their carers exaggerate the pain. Murray and May (1988) report that one-third of their respondents with SCD reported long delays in hospitals and not receiving adequate pain relief. For instance, patients in severe pain often have to wait for lengthy periods in accident and emergency departments before being admitted to the wards, during which time they are often seen by inexperienced doctors and asked what they regard as inappropriate questions (Maxwell and Streetly 1998; Atkin and Ahmad 2000a). Mothers of children with an SCD – as we have seen – complain that they cannot trust health professionals with the care of their children (Atkin *et al.* 2000).

Further, stereotypes of minority ethnic patients having a lower pain threshold are rife in the health services (Ahmad *et al.* 1991; Bowler 1993) and may influence treatment of pain. Health professionals, for example, often feel those with SCD are overreacting and exaggerating their pain (Atkin *et al.* 1998a). The lack of treatment can also be justified by another racial myth. Some people with SCD require powerful drugs for the control of pain. However, some doctors worry about their black patients becoming dependent on drugs (Stimmel 1983; Ballas 1990) and this can contribute to the significant undertreatment of pain. There is no evidence to suggest that addiction to powerful pain-killing drugs is a significant problem among SCD sufferers (Midence and Elander 1994). More generally, as Hurtig (1994) has pointed out, the medical myth is that pain in SCD is 'manipulative', and can 'serve to demand attention at best and drugs at worst'. This contributes to the poor pain relief available to people during a painful crisis and means that one of the most distressing aspects of their illness remains poorly treated (Department of Health 1993; Maxwell *et al*. 1999).

For their part, health professionals and managers often admit there are problems in providing pain relief (Atkin *et al*. 1998a; Maxwell and Streetly 1998). They recognize, for example, that the racial myths held by frontline practitioners often deny pain relief when it is needed. They are also aware that some ward staff do not appreciate the severity of pain because they do not have a general understanding of SCD (Atkin *et al*. 1998a, 1998b). Even protocols for pain relief, often introduced as a response to the Standing Medical Advisory Committee (SMAC) report (Department of Health 1993), are not followed as a consequences of these difficulties (Atkin *et al*. 1998a).

The problem in treating pain is particularly unfortunate since individuals and their families described it as the worst aspect of living with SCD (see previous chapter). The inability of services to deal with pain contributes to the vulnerability of individuals and their families and means they remain unsupported during one of the most difficult and demanding times of their life. To underline a point made in the previous chapter, health professionals rather than offering care become part of the problem and add to the difficulties of living with an SCD.

Thalassaemia and blood transfusions

For thalassaemia major, availability of beds for monthly transfusions remains a problem in some localities (Darr 1990; Anionwu 1993). Patients and their families are also unhappy about the time spent waiting before the transfusion goes ahead (Anionwu 1996a) and the occasional difficulties they face because of inexperienced staff who are not knowledgeable about the transfusion process (Atkin and Ahmad 2000b). Other difficulties include the timing of transfusions (Darr 1997). Parents, for example, often have to take time off work to accompany children and would prefer transfusions to take place in the evenings or at weekends. Young children and adults would support this, so as to ensure that blood transfusions did not disrupt education or employment. Some areas offer flexible provision and this is appreciated by both individuals and families (Madgwick and Yardumian 1999). This flexibility, however, is not available in some areas (Atkin *et al*. 1998a, 2000). The cost of regular transport to hospitals may also cause problems for some families, particularly if they have a low income (Darr 1990; Anionwu 1993). These problems can contribute to the vulnerability of coping strategies (see previous chapter). Further, young people and parents often complain about a lack of information on and support with chelation therapy (Atkin *et al*. 1998a; Atkin and Ahmad 2000c). More generally, some families often lack basic information about how to care for an affected child (Atkin *et al*. 1998a).

Communication and service support

The lack of interpreting and translating services within the NHS compounds the problems faced by Asian families caring for a child with thalassaemia (Darr 1990; Butt 1994; ALG 2000) and represents another example of institutional racism, in which diversity is not recognized (Walker and Ahmad 1994). Sometimes family members are used as interpreters and, although acceptable to some parents, others objected to the practice (Atkin *et al.* 1998a). In some cases young children are required to act as interpreters of complex medical information, often about sensitive or potentially embarrassing issues (Atkin *et al.* 1998b). Young people, for example, often withheld information from their parents. Sometimes this is to protect the parents, at other times, however, it is to disguise their non-compliance with medical regimens (Atkin and Ahmad 2000c). Mothers also pointed to the problems their husband faced in simultaneously translating distressing information and coming to terms with it themselves (Atkin *et al.* 1998a). Fathers confirm these problems and had particular difficulties in deciding how much they should tell their non-English speaking wives; often they wanted to 'protect' them from information deemed upsetting. However this often left mothers without important information about thalassaemia – information important for understanding, coping and caring. This is especially significant because these mothers usually took on the main responsibility of care, yet were dependent on another gatekeeper for information about the condition. This contrasts with the situation of mothers whose children had SCD; they had direct contact with practitioners (Atkin *et al.* 2000). Consequently, many Asian mothers were left without a 'voice' and this is why specialist haemoglobinopathy workers who shared the linguistic and cultural background of these women were especially valued.[1] We discuss this issue in more detail below.

Difficulties still occur when interpreters are used (Chamba *et al.* 1998). Most interpreters, for example, had little specialist knowledge about thalassaemia and faced difficulties in interpreting clinical information and procedures, sometimes with unfortunate consequences (Atkin *et al.* 1998a). This meant that parents often gained misleading and erroneous information about their child's illness. Atkin *et al.* (1998a) cite an example of one family who did not realize thalassaemia was a genetic condition until after the birth of their third child with the condition. Previous translators had simply said the child was born with the condition. Families also point to the problems of communicating through a third party. This, they felt, made it difficult to ask questions and more generally take part in a discussion with health professionals. Not surprisingly, families are dissatisfied with the process (Katbamna *et al.* 1997; Atkin *et al.* 1998b; Chamba *et al.* 1999).

Many practitioners share these concerns about the shortfalls in interpreting services (Atkin *et al.* 1998b). For example, interpreters were often not available or else difficult to organize. For these reasons, many health professionals preferred to use family members (Atkin *et al.* 1998b). Even when interpreting services are available, practitioners still identified problems. Several practitioners remarked that there were often differences in the language or dialect spoken by the interpreter and that spoken by the patient. Others questioned interpreters' skills in translating genetic information as well as their own competence in working with interpreters (Chamba *et al.* 1998). Many health professionals, for example, are not trained in using interpreters, and found this a barrier to effective communication (Atkin *et al.* 1998b).

Health professionals recognized, however, that barriers to communications were more than language specific and evoke cultural differences (Walker and Ahmad 1994), particularly since the racial myths and stereotypes can corrupt the communication process. Darr (1990), for example, notes that in relation to thalassaemia major in the Pakistani community, health professionals often related the condition explicitly (and less often implicitly) to consanguineous marriages and therefore considered it to be self-inflicted. The relationship between consanguineous marriage and the incidence of genetic conditions is complex (Ahmad *et al.* 2000). Nonetheless, associating thalassaemia with first-cousin marriages informs part of the general discourse about the condition and as such can have implications for self-image, provoking resentfulness and guilt (Ahmad *et al.* 2000). Health professionals' focus on first-cousin marriage also appears to be at the expense of providing other, perhaps more important information. Despite their generally poor understanding of thalassaemia, its treatment and consequences for their child, many parents thought it was 'caused' by first-cousin marriage, largely a reflection of what they had been told by professionals (Atkin *et al.* 1998b). More generally the emphasis on consanguineous marriage among health professionals is seen by some commentators as an example of the implicit racism in medical discourse, in which the health problems of people from ethnic minorities become located in their presumed cultural and biological pathology (Ahmad 1996b; Darr 1997).

Except for specialist haemoglobinopathy workers, most professionals feel ill-equipped to respond to cultural differences (Dyson 1998; Atkin *et al.* 1998b). This reflects their own lack of training, which means they are unable to meet the needs of minority ethnic groups (Ahmad 1993). Specialist workers' understanding of cultural perspectives and their language skills, however, helped them offer better tailored information and culturally appropriate support (Anionwu 1996b; Atkin *et al.* 1998b). Mothers particularly appreciated being able to talk to someone who shared their own gender – especially important considering these mothers were often marginalized during the process of service delivery (Atkin *et al.* 1998b).

Building on examples of good practice

Despite the many problems faced by individuals and their families, examples of good practice do exist. We have already seen how specialist haemoglobinopathy workers or counsellors provide important support for families by sharing the same linguistic and cultural background. More generally these workers are identified as fundamental in offering individuals and their families coordinated service provision (Anionwu 1996b). These workers are particularly valued for their practical advice as well as social and emotional support (Atkin *et al.* 2000). The nature of support also means that these workers have ongoing contact with families and this enabled them to develop rapport and trust. Perhaps not surprisingly, individuals and their families say these workers are often the most valuable contact they have, many times restoring their confidence in NHS provision. Atkin *et al.* (2000) for example report parents' comments such as 'guardian angel', 'a godsend', 'I don't know what I would do without her', when discussing their view of these specialist workers. More generally, specialist workers are fundamental in ensuring families' needs are met, often making up for deficiencies they experience elsewhere in the NHS (Anionwu 1996b).

Families and individuals also describe positive relationships with some consultants and other health professionals (Atkin *et al.* 1998a, 2000; Maxwell and Streetly 1998; Atkin and Ahmad 2000b). Particular attributes valued by affected individuals and their families include medical competence, approachability, an ability to listen, an understanding of their situation and putting them at their ease. This offers another reminder that general services can be sensitive to the needs of individuals and their families.

Social care, benefits, and interagency collaboration

Besides health care provision, young people and their parents also experience problems with other agencies. Individuals and their families, for instance, have little contact with social service departments (SSDs), and, for their part, SSDs do not see haemoglobinopathies as a priority because they were reluctant to seek out another area of unmet need (Atkin *et al.* 1998a). This, however, seems in contrast to other forms of chronic illness (Beresford *et al.* 1996), where social workers have more of a commitment to meet the needs of individuals and families (Baldwin and Carlisle 1994).

The role of social care agencies is also disregarded in policy guidance, as it is assumed haemoglobinopathies are a health care issue. The risks of disability that these conditions can cause, as set out in Chapters 2 and 3, are not widely known by social care practitioners. The otherwise extensive guidance produced by the SMAC Report (Department of Health 1993), for example, virtually ignored the role of social services, housing and education services in supporting families. This is despite evidence suggesting there is an important role for social services in supporting the needs of individuals and their families (Nash 1977, 1994; LePontois 1986; Evans 1988). Potential support, for example, could include the provision of information, assessment of need, advice, guidance and counselling, and provision of occupational, social, cultural and recreational activities.

The previous chapter also suggested the housing agencies can help support individuals with a haemoglobinopathy. Their response, however, is often ill-informed with local authorities and housing associations having little understanding about the consequences of haemoglobinopathies (Black and Laws 1986). This meant those with a haemoglobinopathy find their housing needs are not given sufficient priority (Anionwu 1993) and this, especially in the case of SCD, exacerbates the symptoms of their illness (Midence and Elander 1994).

Families and individuals also experience problems with the Department of Social Security, which is criticized for failing to understand the cost implications of haemoglobinopathies (Atkin *et al.* 1998a, 2000). The Department of Social Security is also criticized for not understanding the consequences of living with a haemoglobinopathy (Black and Laws 1986). This means that many individuals, for example, are often turned down for Disability Living Allowance on spurious grounds, which reflects the ignorance of the assessor rather than the needs of the individual (Atkin *et al.* 2000). Assessors, for example, sometimes confuse the condition with the trait. More generally, assessors seem unaware of the complications associated with haemoglobinopathies, their unpredictable onset and the possible limitations imposed by the illness. Perhaps not surprisingly, individuals and their families feel it is a struggle to get help with the financial costs of their illness. This confirms more general literature suggesting that disability benefits are poorly targeted and their allocation arbitrary.

Interagency collaboration is also poor, with little joint working between primary and secondary health care providers, as well as between health care providers and education authorities, social services and other agencies (Atkin *et al.* 1998a; Ahmad and Atkin 2000). Parents, for example, identify this lack of coordination as a particular problem in ensuring their child receives adequate care, and not surprisingly, wanted a single accessible source of comprehensive information (Atkin and Ahmad 2000a). Like many family caregivers, parents favour a key worker who can provide support and advice as well as coordinate the services parents need (see Glendinning 1985 for a more detailed discussion of the value of a key worker). This is also relevant for adult provision (Anionwu 1996b). To some extent – as we have seen – specialist haemoglobinopathy counsellors fulfil this role and are highly valued by parents and those with the condition (Atkin *et al.* 1998a, 1998b). This further underlines the importance of such workers in providing support to individuals and their families. Unfortunately, not all individuals and their families have access to a haemoglobinopathy counsellor and there are considerable regional variations in their distribution (Anionwu 1996a; Atkin *et al.* 1998a).

Haemoglobinopathies and education

Education, although only having an immediate effect on young people and their families, can have far reaching implications. Interruptions to schooling are a particular difficulty facing children with haemoglobinopathies and a general feature of growing up with a chronic illness (Mador and

Smith 1989; Davis and Wasserman 1992; Wjst *et al.* 1996). School attendance, for example, can be disrupted by painful crisis in SCD (Walco and Dampier 1990) or the need for regular blood transfusions in thalassaemia (Darr 1990). Further, both SCD and thalassaemia make demands on the children that may, in the short term, have to take priority over education (Shapiro *et al.* 1995). Consequently affected children could lose out academically and become isolated from friends and peers (Conyard *et al.* 1980). Regular school attendance and participation, for example, are essential elements in the children's intellectual and social development and psychosocial well-being (Nash 1990; Midence and Elander 1994; Fuggle *et al.* 1996). In addition to formal education, school provides opportunities for leisure as well as social interaction with peers. When things go wrong for children at school, the personal and social development and overall quality of life may be reduced significantly (Fowler *et al.* 1986; Fuggle *et al.* 1996). Academic achievement is also important because the restrictions and limitations of sickle cell disorders and thalassaemia may make manual jobs untenable. Qualifications may afford people with greater opportunity to seek work compatible with their condition (Nettles 1994).

Parents and young people experience many problems with schooling (Anionwu 1992; Atkin *et al.* 2000). Evidence from North America suggests this lack of understanding of the condition on the part of schools, creates many difficulties for young people during their school careers, often meaning they do not fulfil their potential (Shapiro *et al.* 1995; Fuggle *et al.* 1996). More generally, families and individuals describe education services as unresponsive to their needs (Anionwu 1993; Midence and Elander 1994). It is to these problems we now turn. Most young people felt their illness had affected their academic progress (Atkin and Ahmad 2000b), although they actively attempted to overcome the disruptions caused by their illness and engaged friends, parents and teachers to help them in this. Parents were especially important in attempting to overcome these disruptions (Fuggle *et al.* 1996). Overcoming disruption to schooling, however, was far from easy and often the school did not seem to offer much support (Atkin and Ahmad 2000b). Young people became annoyed when they felt that teachers had 'written off' their chances of academic success (Shapiro *et al.* 1995). Schools were particularly criticized for not being proactive in providing extra work to catch up, despite the requests of young people and their parents (Atkin and Ahmad 2000a).

The response of teachers especially disappointed young people and made them question their own efforts (Atkin and Ahmad 2000b). Young people, for instance, remarked that there were times when they lost interest in education as a consequence of their illness (Midence and Elander 1994). This seemed more likely to happen when the child was between 13 and 15 years old, and was particularly common among boys (Atkin and Ahmad 2000b, 2000c). These young people found it difficult to keep up or did not see the point of school. Young boys became especially disruptive and angry. Generally, this is a further illustration of the vulnerability of young people's coping strategies discussed in the previous chapter. Schools, however, do not seem to recognize this (Midence and Elander 1994).

Another problem faced by parents and young people concerned the inability of teachers to deal with medical problems and potential medical crises at school (Midence and Elander 1994). Young people, for example, had little confidence that their teachers would be able to cope if they fell ill at school and this worried them. Parents shared these concerns and commented on the ignorance of many teachers, who often felt the child exaggerated the consequences of the illness (Atkin *et al.* 1998a). What especially annoyed parents was that they made many efforts to educate teachers but felt their efforts were constantly ignored. Parents, for instance, said teachers disregarded their instructions and made their child take part in activities which could prove harmful to the child's health (Hill 1994). Examples often cited by parents and affected children in Britain include an insistence on strenuous sporting activities and staying out in the playground in very cold, windy and damp weather conditions. The educational needs of children with disabilities (such as following a stroke in a child with SCD) requires greater study.

Finally, few young people had received what they regarded as helpful careers advice at school (Atkin and Ahmad 2000b), despite it being especially important for those with a chronic illness (Nettles 1994). Careers advisers do not seem well informed about haemoglobinopathies and young people did not see career advice as helpful in deciding what their careers options were. In some cases the involvement of the careers adviser was especially negative (Atkin and Ahmad 2000c). Several young people commented that the careers adviser had especially low expectations of the young person's ability. Careers officers' indifference, however, was sometimes attributed to racism, reflecting a more general problem (Braham *et al.* 1992). Older Asian girls, for instance, felt that careers officers did not expect them to pursue a career, while African-Caribbean young people felt that careers officers had predetermined ideas about the types of work they could do. This offers another example of how racism adds to the difficulties of those with a haemoglobinopathy.

The development of haemoglobinopathy provision

Calls for better coordination of services both at the local as well as national level have repeatedly been made by some health workers (Franklin 1988; Davies *et al.* 1993; Streetly *et al.* 1993; Davies 1994), patients' organizations (Sickle Cell Society 1981) and official working parties (Department of Health 1993; Health Education Authority 1998). One welcome development, and a useful model for developing coordinated services, is the increasing network of haemoglobinopathy counselling centres since the very first one was established in 1979 in Brent (Anionwu 1989). Employing specialist haemoglobinopathy workers, these centres combine services such as information, screening, educational courses for both community members and professionals as well as advice about other services and benefits. As we have seen, specialist workers employed in these centres are praised by individuals and families for the support they offer. Such workers offer linguistically and culturally sensitive support in local community settings and are able to facilitate successful interagency collaboration (Anionwu 1996a; Atkin *et al.* 1998a, 1998b; Gould *et al.* 2000). More generally, such workers are recognized as significantly improving the provision of information, screening, genetic counselling and support services for those at risk of haemoglobinopathies (World Health Organization 1988; Royal College of Physicians 1989). A former consultant haematologist in the West Midlands noted that:

> Sickle cell counsellors have been of immense value in providing support and advice for patients and their families and education and screening for the community. They are also ideally placed to tackle educational and employment problems in both the school and work place.
>
> (Franklin 1988: 592)

A study undertaken in 1995 identified that 37 districts employed 57 sickle cell and thalassaemia counsellors, the vast majority of whom were minority ethnic nurses and midwives (Anionwu 1996a). The growth in haemoglobinopathy centres has been encouraging, though many would argue still inadequately resourced (Anionwu 1993; Potrykus 1993; Gould *et al.* 2000). Nonetheless, such centres represent an important starting point in developing haemoglobinopathy provision and provide the potential for empowering people from minority ethnic groups, discussed in more detail in the final chapter.

More generally, the impact of all this policy interest in haemoglobinopathies, however, has yet to be evaluated and various difficulties exist. Not least is their advisory nature and the lack of any allocation of resources to fund the various recommendations made by reports. This has led some critics to question the impact of the SMAC report, despite the excellence of many of its recommendations (Davies 1994; Streetly *et al.* 1997). We have seen, for example, that although protocols for pain relief have been established in response to the report (Department of Health 1993), there is no guarantee they will be used by frontline staff (see Maxwell *et al.* 1999). Further, Chapter 4 documented a range of problems in providing screening and counselling services. The unsatisfactory transfer of care from paediatric to adult services remains another difficulty (Davies *et al.* 1993) despite the existence of policy and practice guidance. Often, for instance, there is little preparation for the transfer and communication between health professionals is generally poor. Young people's emotional concerns about the transition are often not dealt with (Atkin and Ahmad 2000b); addressing their concerns is important, particularly since it has taken them many years to establish rapport and trust with their previous health professionals. Generally, the transfer from children to adult services increases the problems experienced by young people and their families at what is already a stressful time (Telfair 1994).

Primary health care remains on the margins of haemoglobinopathy provision despite its potential importance in providing screening, as well as support to families and individuals (Department of Health 1993; Modell *et al.* 1998; Ahmad and Atkin 2000). Few individuals and families, however, have regular contact with members of the primary health care team and do not see a role for GPs or other members of the primary health care team in the management of their illness (Darr 1990; Midence and Elander 1994; Maxwell and Streetly 1998; Ahmad and Atkin 2000). They prefer to rely on their consultant, who they felt knew more about the condition (Ahmad and Atkin 2000; Atkin *et al.* 2000). Primary health care staff agree with individuals and families and feel that hospital staff and specialist workers are in a better position to offer support (Ahmad and Atkin 2000). Hospital staff and health commissioners, however, would prefer greater involvement of GPs in haemoglobinopathy provision, but are not sure how this can be achieved (Ahmad and Atkin 2000). Coordinating general practice, as well as the considerable variations in the quality of primary health care provision, were identified as particular problems (Ahmad and Atkin 2000).

The management and organization of haemoglobinopathy provision raises more generic problems (Davies *et al.* 1993). As we have seen, specialist workers often act as guarantors of good practice. They, however, often work in NHS Trusts who do not always understand their role or the importance of community development (Potrykus 1991; Anionwu 1996a; Atkin *et al.* 1998a; Gould *et al.* 2000). There seemed, for example, to be a constant tension between the work of the specialist worker and their managers about the scope of the workers' role. Trust managers were keen to concentrate on the more medical aspects of the workers' role. This reflects a more general concern of health care agencies to draw boundaries around their own role and distinguish between a health and social care need (Twigg 1997). The reluctance of social care agencies to offer support to individuals and their families suggests that haemoglobinopathy provision would be further undermined by making specialist workers focus on health care needs and reduce the social support they offer. At present there is no one to take their place, especially since social service departments do not regard haemoglobinopathies as a priority (Anionwu 1996a; Atkin *et al.* 1998a).

Specialist haemoglobinopathy workers are also located outside mainstream NHS clinical genetic centres (Anionwu 1993). This contrasts with workers providing genetic counselling for other illnesses such as cystic fibrosis. Some argue this situation will further marginalize haemoglobinopathy provision, resulting in continuing low status and inadequate funding (Anionwu 1996a). The specialist workers themselves seem to be aware of these problems and complain that the current services represent a token gesture on behalf of health care agencies to meet the needs of minority ethnic groups (Atkin *et al.* 1998a). These workers, despite the valuable support they offer, often believe they are marginalized within their organization and not taken seriously (Potrykus 1993; Anionwu 1996a). They are also subject to the same racism that affects their other black colleagues working in the NHS (Beishon *et al*. 1995; Gerrish *et al*. 1996).

Specialist workers specifically criticize health authorities for failing to take a strategic lead on developing haemoglobinopathy provision (Atkin *et al*. 1998a). Health authority managers agree that this is a problem and rarely monitor or audit contracts (Atkin *et al*. 1998b). This problem, although not unique to haemoglobinopathy provision (Office of Public Management 1996), means that the health authority managers have little knowledge about the service provided and therefore could not influence service development. Again this is not unique to haemoglobinopathy services (Flynn *et al*. 1996), but could mean that an already marginal service was further neglected. The inability to evaluate haemoglobinopathy provision was also caught up in the general difficulties faced by health care agencies in ensuring equal opportunities. Trust and health authority managers are aware that minority ethnic groups face disadvantage and discrimination, but point to the difficulties of achieving change, despite a formal commitment to equal opportunities (Atkin and Rollings 1993). There is no doubting this commitment to change and many care agencies are trying to offer more sensitive provision (Butt 1994). Few equal opportunity policies, however, are monitored and are often criticized for being a paper exercise with little commitment to change (Butt 1994). The final chapter will explore the opportunities raised by the publication of the Equal Opportunities Framework for the National Health Service (NHSE 2000).

Nonetheless, the requirement that health authorities plan services on the basis of health needs assessment can potentially be an effective vehicle for getting haemoglobinopathies on the agenda (Ahmad 1993). Health commissioners are aware of this and also point to the importance of lobbying and community action. This is an especially important point given the scope of this book. Health commissioners, for example, admit that services often go to those who shout loudest (Atkin *et al*. 1998a). To this extent, the extensive guidance proposed by the Standing Medical Advisory Committee (Department of Health 1993) and other documents (Modell and Anionwu 1996; Health Education Authority 1998) could be used by communities and commissioners alike to effect change. Other writers (Walker and Ahmad 1994) note the general importance of this for minority ethnic groups. These authors argue that despite the many disadvantages facing minority ethnic groups, they need to exploit existing mechanisms and policy opportunities to ensure their voice is heard in developing appropriate and accessible service provision. Various ideas for future strategies are explored in the final chapter.

Nonetheless, it should be stated that many local and national organizations have attempted to take advantage of this increased policy interest in haemoglobinopathies. Indeed, as we have seen, in many areas the development of haemoglobinopathy provision was the direct consequence of community action, often over many years, in which at risk communities defined their own needs and brought them to the attention of those responsible for organizing services (Anionwu 1988). Active community pressure, for instance, was responsible for the first sickle cell counselling centre being established in the UK in 1979 (Anionwu 1993) and this model was soon followed in other urban areas (Anionwu 1996a). Examples included Manchester, Liverpool, Birmingham and Cardiff (Manchester Community Health Group 1981; Torkington 1983; Franklin 1988; Choiseul *et al.* 1988) as well as other London boroughs (Prashar *et al.* 1985; Black and Laws 1986). Change on the basis of community action, therefore, is possible (Beattie 1986; Hogg 1999). Nonetheless, there is also some disillusionment, particularly among local groups, at the lack of political will and non-recognition of need by health and social care agencies. These local groups, for example, often feel they should not have to fight for a service when the need for one is obvious (see Barnardo's 1993). This is characteristic of the relationship between minority ethnic voluntary sector and mainstream agencies (Atkin 1996). Nonetheless, the importance of this type of local organization should not be underestimated and they have been central in securing haemoglobinopathy provision in the UK and to this extent provide a positive example of black empowerment (Stuart 1996). Their influence needs to continue.

Besides local organizations, national organizations, such as the Sickle Cell Society, Organisation for Sickle Cell Anaemia Research (OSCAR) and UK Thalassaemia Society, continue the struggle to secure appropriate and accessible haemoglobinopathy provision (Anionwu 1993) and also to provide other successful examples of black empowerment. These organizations offer important social and emotional support for individuals and families, provide information and advice as well as lobby for improved provision. They have also begun to secure funding to develop provision for individuals and their families. The UK Thalassaemia Society, for example, has secured National Lottery funding to improve knowledge of thalassaemia among Asian families. The Sickle Cell Society continues to develop local services such as peer counselling, home tutorial provision and respite support. OSCAR has developed many thriving local groups in areas such as the West Midlands, Reading, Bristol and south London. Their contribution is greatly appreciated by individuals and their families (Darr 1990; Anionwu 1996a; Atkin *et al.* 1998a, 1998b) and they play an important role in the politics of sickle cell and thalassaemia. We will return to their role in the final chapter when we consider the potential for strategy and struggle.

Conclusion

This chapter reviewed the role of health and social care agencies in providing services to individuals and families with a haemoglobinopathy. The chapter paints a bleak picture, with haemoglobinopathy provision appearing erratic, lacking in coordination and unable to meet the needs of individuals and their families. Consequently, those with a haemoglobinopathy and their families receive inadequate and poor quality support that denies even the most basic care needs. These problems reflect the more general difficulties facing minority ethnic people in having their health and social care needs recognized and catered for. As we have argued throughout the book, haemoglobinopathy provision is caught up in the general struggle for more equitable provision faced by minority ethnic groups.

Specific shortfalls include inadequate information, unsupportive, unsympathetic and poorly informed service providers and teachers, inappropriate treatment, racist assumptions informing attitudes of some staff, insensitivity to the individuals' and families' worries, and failure to meet their needs. The problems occur across health and social care agencies. This in itself is a reminder that haemoglobinopathies are not simply a health care issue. Social services, housing agencies, the benefits agency and education services have an important role in supporting those with a haemoglobinopathy and their families.

Rectifying the general difficulties faced by individuals and their families becomes an important focus for strategy and struggle aimed at improving haemoglobinopathy provision. The increasing importance of needs assessment and a more user-centred service system offers a potential lever for change. It is also important to build on current examples of good practice. Individuals' high regard for specialist workers and some other health professionals reminds us, however, that services can be sensitive. There are more general examples of service delivery in which many of the difficulties faced by individuals and their families have been successfully dealt with. Examples of good practice do exist and it is important that these influence current provision, providing models for empowerment. As part of this, community action and voluntary organizations – both local and national – have played an important role in establishing and improving current provision. In some areas, for example, there would be little or no provision without the activities of these organizations, who also continue to provide valuable support and advice to individuals and their families. This provides an important example of black empowerment and self-help, illustrating the importance of community activity grounded in critical insight. Such organizations will continue to be central in the development of sickle cell and thalassaemia provision. The final chapter explores the potential for change in greater detail and looks towards the future.

Note

1 There is no consistency in job titles among those who are employed by the NHS to work specifically on SCD and thalassaemia. Common titles include 'haemoglobinopathy counsellor', 'haemoglobinopathy project worker', 'nurse specialist', 'health promotion nurse specialist' or 'outreach nurse'. For simplicity, the book refers to these workers as 'specialist workers'.

7

Past achievements and future strategies

In this book, we have explored the politics of sickle cell and thalassaemia provision in the UK by focusing on two interrelated themes. First, we have charted the significant milestones in understanding the nature, prevalence and management of sickle and thalassaemia disorders. Second, we have explored the impact on individuals and families and discussed the degree to which agencies such as the NHS respond to their needs. In doing so, we have accorded primacy to the views of the patient and their families and demonstrated how future developments need to be grounded in their experience. However, the book, as should be apparent by now, is not just about haemoglobinopathies, but addresses more general policy interests. Recent policy documents, for example, emphasize the need for a more systematic approach to planning and providing culturally sensitive services (see Chamba *et al*. 1999), particularly since there is increasing awareness of how inaccessible and inappropriate provision denies minority ethnic communities adequate care and support (see Ahmad and Atkin 1996a; Acheson 1998).

Empowerment and struggle in improving the lives of minority ethnic communities becomes a unifying theme in linking haemoglobinopathies with these broader concerns. Our narrative shows that despite considerable barriers, progress has been achieved due to a mixture of community and professional action, exerting political pressure on the relevant agencies. To this extent, many of the improvements in the provision of sickle cell and thalassaemia services have occurred as a consequence of these pressures rather than proactive initiatives by health and social care organizations (Atkin *et al*. 1998a, 2000). As part of this, the greater awareness of SCD among the African-Caribbean community – compared to the limited awareness of thalassaemia among the Asian groups (see France-Dawson 1990; Dyson *et al*. 1993; Dyson 1997; Lakhani 1999) – can be traced back to the political activity of the 1980s (Anionwu 1993). The 1990s witnessed a significant amount of interest in the condition as a result of campaigns involving specialized health professionals, local and national sickle cell support groups, a dynamic black voluntary sector, politicians and celebrities.

Despite a sometimes hostile and unsupportive external environment, such community action on haemoglobinopathies offers an example of positive achievement and is a reminder of what struggle and emancipatory activity can accomplish. Future strategies need to build on this and although much has been accomplished, there is considerable work to be done before haemoglobinopathies receive the recognition and resources they deserve. This is part of a continuing struggle – at a national and local level – in which priorities have to be justified.

Future challenges

Various factors will inform current and future struggles. Generally, the continued failure to address institutionalized racism within welfare provision has created an environment that allows inequalities and discrimination in health and social care to go unchallenged (see Beishon *et al.* 1995; Blakemore and Drake 1996; Law 1996; Collier 1999; *Lancet* 1999). This, as we have seen, has been a significant feature in past struggles and has meant the NHS has been extremely slow to recognize haemoglobinopathies as significant public health issues (Anionwu 1996b). Consequently, inadequate, ill coordinated and poorly resourced services continue to present major problems for people with a haemoglobinopathy and their families. Minority ethnic health care workers have to work within a similar racist environment. In this respect, many community and hospital-based haemoglobinopathy specialist workers are minority ethnic nurses and they have found it difficult to obtain high level support concerning their grievances about services starved of resources (Potrykus 1993; Anionwu 1996b). Further, the initial successes, such as the development of sickle cell and thalassaemia counselling centres, ironically led to the belief that haemoglobinopathies 'have been sorted out' and that there was therefore no further need to keep the issue high on the NHS agenda (Anionwu 1993; also see Chapter 6). This is a general problem facing minority ethnic groups, in which one-off gestures on the part of health and social care agencies are seen to solve problems once and for all (see Atkin and Rollings 1996). Regrettably there is often little ongoing commitment.

Institutional racism pervades the entire debate and informs the more specific challenges facing those struggling for better provision. In the first instance, the complexity of changes within the NHS where the commissioner/provider divide led to competitive behaviour for funding and control of services between the acute and community sectors within the same locality is worth noting (Anionwu 1996a). It is difficult to see how the introduction of primary health care groups will improve the situation (see Ahmad and Atkin 2000; Modell *et al.* 2000a). The struggle between various organizations within the NHS has impacted negatively on the ability to organize comprehensive care and screening and counselling services for conditions such as haemoglobinopathies that spanned the territories of various agencies (Atkin *et al*. 1998a, 1998b). Fragmentation thus occurs and at its worse, haemoglobinopathies become someone else's problem.

The lack of leadership shown by national agencies such as the Department of Health and the former Health Education Authority (now replaced by the Health Development Agency) compounds these difficulties. The inability of the Department of Health to give direction, for instance, has resulted in lost opportunities in establishing coherent policy and practice as well as in the funding and facilitating of joint initiatives between the voluntary and statutory sectors. Political pressure from both the UK Thalassaemia Society and the Sickle Cell Society ultimately resulted, in March 2000, in a last minute request from the Department of Health for bids. This enabled, a few days before the end of the financial year, an allocation of funding for both groups to undertake health promotion activities.

The Department of Health remains unsympathetic to professionals campaigning for more central involvement and direction because of their policy of devolving most funding priorities to regional and local health authorities. The exception to this policy was, of course, a core of nationally identified Health of the Nation priorities. As haemoglobinopathies were not included in these priorities it was left to local agencies to determine whether they should be included as additional local priorities. Further, reports on haemoglobinopathy services emanating from the Department of Health (1993) and the Health Education Authority (1998) have had no resources attached, were advisory in nature and therefore offered little, if any, incentive for NHS Trusts and authorities to act upon their recommendations. Local struggles for services still occur throughout the UK and even when services are established some still are vulnerable to short term funding arrangements. The experience of establishing community support in areas such as Sheffield illustrates this, although this should perhaps not surprise us as it is a long standing problem facing voluntary organizations (Atkin 1996). More generally, the lack of clear national policy and practice guidelines is an ongoing problem and it will be of interest to see whether the Department of Health is likely to adopt a more proactive line in the near future. One opportunity may be provided by the Health Development Agency that was established in April 2000 and included in their early priorities is a review of the most appropriate ways of reducing inequalities in health. Having haemoglobinopathies incorporated into Health Improvement Programmes (HImPs) could provide another important opportunity. Both the Health Development Agency and HImP will be discussed further on in the section that identifies opportunities that exist for improving haemoglobinopathy services.

Ineffectual leadership and an inability to make haemoglobinopathies a priority is also reflected in the response of local authorities and the Department of Social Security. Not only do social services, housing, social security and education departments have little understanding of haemoglobinopathies

(Ahmad and Atkin 1996b), they are reluctant to provide support to individuals or families affected by the conditions (Atkin *et al.* 2000). Social security officers regularly confuse SCDs with sickle cell trait and benefits are often refused as a consequence of the assessors' ignorance (Black and Laws 1986; Atkin *et al.* 1998a). Housing departments are guilty of similar errors and often fail to recognize the significance of haemoglobin disorders when making housing decisions (Black and Laws 1986). The development by Enfield and Haringey HA of local authority housing guidelines for people with SCD, however, has been cited as an example of good practice (ALG 2000) and this could provide a valuable resource for other housing agencies. Educational provision is also ill equipped to meet the needs of children and their families (Midence and Elander 1994; Atkin *et al.* 2000). As a consequence children with a sickle cell disorder or thalassaemia experience greater difficulties in securing a 'good' education in comparison to their peers without a chronic illness. Social services, despite the provision of the Children Act, still fail to make adequate provision for those with a haemoglobinopathy disorder, often regarding sickle cell and thalassaemia as a *health* and not a *social care* problem (Atkin *et al.* 1998a).

In addition to the involvement of statutory agencies, the effective organization of the voluntary sector will remain a key to future success. Despite considerable achievements, the role of the voluntary sector can, however, be best described as only being intermittently effective. The 1980s and 1990s, for example, have witnessed fluctuations in the degree of influence that sickle cell and thalassaemia groups have been able to exert at a national level. Campaigning activities in respect to SCD (see Sickle Cell Society 1981) made a significant impression in the 1980s, a fact recognized by Pinder (1985) who cited the Sickle Cell Society as an example of a successful organization. McNaught (1987) agreed and suggested the Society was probably one of the better known minority ethnic health initiatives.

Since the first national sickle cell association (OSCAR) was established in 1975, at least five other national groups have at various times been set up, resulting in fragmentation and diminution of hard won political influence. Fund-raising potential has also been weakened as funding bodies are either unsure of who to support or use the situation to divide and rule. These circumstances also provide an opportunity to justify awarding little or no money to any of the groups.

Confusion and exasperation felt by affected families, community groups and committed professionals was articulated in 1993 at a conference (Barnardo's 1993) aimed at developing collaboration among the various groups. The degree of support for such an objective was demonstrated by the overwhelming attendance of over 500 adults and 110 children and young people. The conference began by recognizing that there had been achievements, but concerns were expressed that increasing fragmentation could undermine this success: 'Ten years ago we didn't have the work we have today . . . We need to encourage ourselves because at least something is being done . . . We need to pool our resources together to help ourselves' (cited in Barnardo's 1993). One delegate articulated the lack of coherence among the voluntary sector more forcefully: 'I'm very angry at this precise moment . . . The problem why we haven't got the money and resources from the government is because we are not one . . . First we've got to get our own house in order' (cited in Barnardo's 1993).

As a response to some of these problems, Hugh Sheriffe, a Barnardo's community development worker, established the first regional forum, the West Midlands Sickle Cell and Thalassaemia Association comprised of local OSCAR groups, health authority projects, voluntary support groups and interested people from housing, education and Barnardo's (Hugh Sheriffe, personal communication). This model of good practice is in the process of being replicated in the setting up of a London Forum (Sickle Cell Society 2000) and Barnardo's is seriously considering supporting these initiatives by funding facilitator posts for each regional forum.

Both the Sickle Cell Society and OSCAR continue to provide information and support. The Sickle Cell Society, for example, has established an extremely useful source of accessible knowledge via their web page. They have also experimented with schemes such as flexible respite care and a newsletter aimed specifically at young people.

The situation for the thalassaemia voluntary sector differs in some respects to that described for sickle cell groups. There is only one national thalassaemia organization, the UK Thalassaemia Society (UKTS) but, in contrast to the situation for sickle cell, there are fewer thalassaemia groups organized at a local level. The national thalassaemia group has demonstrated some wariness in joining forces with sickle cell groups, partly due to the relatively low number of individuals with thalassaemia nationally and the fear that they may not receive due attention in such an umbrella organization, although relationships are improving. The UKTS has a good record in raising awareness of thalassaemia among communities and professionals. It is also an important source of support for those affected by the illness and their families. Its annual conference, for example, is well attended and offers an excellent forum in which professionals, affected individuals and their families can discuss the illness. Established in 1976 by parents and volunteers from the British Cypriot community it took some time, however, before the UKTS had involvement from representatives of the various Asian communities. The organization has subsequently taken a very proactive stance to improve this situation and, as previously noted, undertook a national survey in 1996 which identified that only 5 per cent of Asian people had heard of thalassaemia (Lakhani 1999). They began to address the latter by a National Lottery funded Asian awareness campaign which has involved an active outreach programme aimed at students and young adults, promotion of thalassaemia in the media as well as a plan for an independent evaluation. Further financial support to continue this initiative was provided by the Department of Health in March 2000.

Despite the good intentions of the project and its obvious value in improving understanding among the British Asian communities, certain pitfalls have occurred, particularly the offence caused in certain quarters concerning the nature of the publicity materials developed. Examples include a poster that states that 'Thalassaemia . . . as Asian as the cobra, and equally deadly. It can kill.' This has managed to be both alarming in tone and potentially offensive in its use of the image of the cobra (which is a symbolic icon of the Hindu god Shiva). Several members of the steering group were particularly upset that they had not even been consulted about the contents of the promotional material and when their subsequent comments were not accepted, resigned in protest. This offers a reminder that the way forward in improving haemoglobinopathy provision is not especially straightforward, even when the voluntary sector takes the initiative.

Achieving change: opportunities and threats

There are still important goals to achieve in improving the quality of comprehensive care to affected individuals, developing the organization of screening and counselling services, increasing public and professional awareness, strengthening the impact of the voluntary sector, increasing the funding of research and ensuring evidence based practice. These goals can only be attained as part of mainstream activities that are aimed at redressing inequalities and institutional racism in the care provided by the NHS and local authorities. The NHS and other agencies must, therefore, ensure national provision of equitable, accessible and culturally sensitive services for those affected by or at risk of haemoglobinopathies. This can only be successfully achieved if they are planned, resourced, delivered and evaluated with realistic, rather than token partnership with the voluntary and specialist sectors.

Opportunities for change, however, do exist. This book, for example, has identified an impressive catalogue of reports containing guidelines and recommendations for improvements in services produced by those working within both the voluntary and statutory sectors over the last few decades. It is useful to be reminded that these publications include: Crawford (1974); Sickle Cell Society (1981); Prashar *et al.* (1985); Black and Laws (1986); British Society of Haematology (1988); Franklin (1988); World Health Organization (1988, 1994); Brozovic and Stephens (1991); Department of Health (1993); British Committee for Standards in Haematology (1994); Davies (1994); Modell and Anionwu (1996); Streetly *et al.* (1997); Bain and Chapman (1998); Health Education Authority (1998); Zeuner *et al.* (1999) and Davies *et al.* (2000) and numerous publications by the authors and their associates. Consequently, there is much to build on and strategies at both a national and local level can be developed utilizing significant opportunities that exist as a result of the successes and the lessons learnt from previous struggles. There is much to be proud of.

Added to this is a changed political climate that has at last forced acceptance that institutionalized racism is relevant for all organizations (Macpherson 1999) including the NHS (Alexander 1999; *Lancet* 1999;

McKenzie 1999). As part of this, the Department of Health has accorded priority to improving access and equity of care together with their expectation that NHS Trusts will attain certain targets in the reduction of discriminatory practices towards staff and patients (National Health Service Executive 1998; Alexander 1999; Department of Health 2000b). An Equal Opportunities Framework for the National Health Service has been published (NHSE 2000). This framework contains among its three strategic equality aims one concerned with recruiting, developing and retaining a workforce that is able to 'deliver high quality services that are accessible, responsive and appropriate to meet the diverse needs of different groups and individuals'. Key actions set out for this aim that could be utilized in better awareness and services for sickle cell and thalassaemia include:

- NHS employers, education consortia and education providers must ensure that the learning environment and curriculum are non-discriminatory and promote understanding and skills to meet the needs of diverse communities;
- service providers must train staff to make sure they understand and keep abreast of the needs of all patient groups;
- service providers must train and support staff to dismantle communication barriers that stop users from getting the services they need.

All NHS organizations will be required to publish an 'equality statement' as part of their annual report outlining for all staff and users how the organization has taken forward national and local priorities and objectives during the year and in its forward plans.

Other more specific Department of Health initiatives may further help improve current provision. In the wake of various screening scandals, and to redress the piecemeal and uncoordinated development of screening policies, the government established the UK National Screening Committee in July 1996. With a remit to advise ministers and their appropriate NHS executive boards, the committee's work embraces the two main themes of policy development and quality management for existing and proposed screening programmes.

Haemoglobinopathies are on the agendas of both the Antenatal and Child Health subgroups and their recommendations are directed to the main national screening committee. There has, however, been confusion about the nature of recommendations made by the Child Health Group and we will explore this further in our discussion on the UK Forum on Haemoglobin Disorders.

Despite this, the issues surrounding screening for sickle cell and thalassaemia have at last been mainstreamed and placed with equal status alongside Down's syndrome, cystic fibrosis and HIV. Issues that are being, or have been, debated include a redefining of the objectives of screening and the development of an overall infrastructure that will be required for any screening programme. These have particular relevance to haemoglobinopathy screening programmes because, as we have seen, the lack of any consensus and authoritative national statement has caused tensions and contributed to the poor quality of service.

An important influence on the deliberations of both the National Screening Committee and the subgroups are the reviews funded by the Population Screening arm of the NHS Health and Technology Assessment (HTA) Programme. Two haemoglobinopathy reviews were included in the portfolio of commissioned projects; other topics have comprised Down's syndrome, HIV, cystic fibrosis, fragile X and ultrasound screening in pregnancy. Both of the two haemoglobinopathy screening reviews have been published (Zeuner *et al.* 1999; Davies *et al.* 2000) and can be accessed through the HTA website. These reviews should help focus debate on national policy and practice together with other sources of UK evidence-based data that can inform the need for improvements and change. Prime examples are the publications from two projects funded from the NHS Research and Development programme, one an evaluation of sickle cell and thalassaemia services in the north of England (Atkin *et al.* 1998a, 1998b), and the second focusing on screening for haemoglobinopathies in primary care (Modell *et al.* 1998). Important information has also emerged from the thalassaemia module of a UK Confidential Enquiry into Counselling for Genetic Disorders (Modell *et al.* 2000a).

Further aspects of how service provision can be refined have been assisted by several London based studies on sickle cell disorders. These have incorporated a needs assessment and estimate of prevalence (Streetly *et al.* 1997), user perspectives concerning pain management (Maxwell *et al.* 1999) and the impact of cognitive behavioural therapy (Thomas *et al.* 1998). Most of these investigations have incorporated a wider perspective than that generally seen in much previous research, which has been more influenced by the traditional medical model. This mixture is encouraging as it can facilitate a more informed debate than previously possible.

The London bias of many of the debates about haemoglobinopathies, however, continues. This is not to see some of the 'London experience' as irrelevant to the UK. The London based studies cited above, for instance, raise issues not specific to the south of England. The experience of pain and its management, for instance, raises generic issues (see Maxwell *et al.* 1999; Atkin and Ahmad 2000b) and there is much that can be learnt about the development of haemoglobinopathy provision in the south of England. Nonetheless, the distribution and make-up of the 'at-risk' populations and the organization of service delivery, which in many areas is less well developed, raise particular issues that have sometimes been neglected in recent national debates.

Such opportunities, suggested by the growing interest in haemoglobinopathy provision do not, however, guarantee change. As we have seen, struggle by communities and proactive engagement by statutory agencies are required. Otherwise, evidence based practice and nationally set guidelines will have little direct impact. Many of the important recommendations made by the Standing Medical Advisory Committee Report in 1993, as we have seen, have failed to find their way into policy and practice. As we have argued in the introduction, focusing on those affected by haemoglobin-opathies is not the same as meeting their needs. Positive action is required once needs have been identified. We have already noted the importance of the voluntary sector in achieving change. Professional groups also have an important role to play and here opportunities present themselves.

The establishment of the UK Forum on Haemoglobin Disorders in 1995 further establishes the possibility for positive change and ensures research findings inform policy and practice. It developed from the London Haemo-globin Disorders Forum, which had previously existed for seven years. The UK Forum is a multidisciplinary group of over 200 people involved in various aspects of sickle cell and thalassaemia services such as haemo-globinopathy counsellors, haematologists, paediatricians, nurses, midwives, medical laboratory scientific staff, obstetricians, representatives from the voluntary sector, public health doctors, psychologists, sociologists, social workers, and molecular geneticists. Their aims include promoting optimal and equitable services for haemoglobin disorders and facilitating collaborat-ive research, developing a network of interdisciplinary contacts and acting as an advisory group to relevant agencies (for an example see Bain and Chapman 1998). In 1995 the UK Forum successfully asked the British Library to include haemoglobinopathies in their MEDLINE Update series (examples included cystic fibrosis and prenatal diagnosis). This is distributed through subscription on a quarterly basis thereby enabling people to be kept up-to-date with the most recent references on sickle cell and thalassaemia.

The Forum organizes two national meetings a year, one in London and the other hosted elsewhere in the UK. The Forum, however, perhaps should take on a more significant leadership role in order to determine changes in the world of sickle cell and thalassaemia services and progress their aim of promoting optimal and equitable care. This will require a proactive stance that ensures that they are aware of the powerful forces with which they must engage to influence and determine policy.

The Forum has demonstrated its ability to do just this by responding to the alarm generated at their May 2000 meeting specifically focusing on the two HTA screening reviews by a speaker from the Child Health Subgroup of the National Screening Committee. The latter had been asked to set out the aims and structure of the National Screening Committee and their subgroups (Antenatal and Child Health) and explain how recommendations from the latter groups that had been agreed by the main committee were then forwarded to ministers for their approval. The example he cited from the Child Health Subgroup concerning haemoglobinopathies was that they recommended that there should be antenatal screening for thalassaemia and neonatal screening for sickle cell disorders. The 200 strong audience was in uproar at the apparent oversight of antenatal screening for sickle cell disorders. Several members of the Antenatal Screening Subgroup were present and were utterly astonished to hear of this apparent development. They were confused as to why the Child Health Subgroup had made a recommendation to do with screening in pregnancy and would take the matter up with their own chairman. The Chairman of the UK Forum on Haemoglobin Disorders received unanimous support for the proposal that he write to the Secretary of State for Health, on behalf of the Forum, to express concern and for clarification at what appears to be a retrograde step. Of tremendous significance is that the NHS Plan, published in July 2000, announced that by the year 2004 there will be 'a new national linked antenatal and neonatal screening programme for haemoglobinopathy and sickle cell disease (Department of Health 2000b: 109).

It is also crucial that a body like the UK Forum has a keen awareness of the wider forces impacting on the future reconfiguration and priorities of health and social agencies, a prime example being the Health Improvement Programmes (HImPs) that each health authority is required to produce for their local population (Department of Health 1997). Many of the strategic themes that form the basis of HImPs have a particular relevance for sickle and thalassaemia services and include:

• public health and inequalities in health;
• the range and location of health and relevant social services;
• the national framework for assessing performance; and
• involving patients and the public in planning and monitoring services.

The UK Forum in conjunction with health care agencies and the voluntary sector needs to determine how haemoglobinopathies are to be included on the agendas of local HImPs. A current example of good practice is the success of the expert haemoglobinopathy working group in west London in respect to ensuring inclusion of forward planning for services into the HImP for Ealing, Hammersmith and Hounslow Health Authority (EHHA). SCD and thalassaemia have been incorporated into the Health Inequalities section and include developments such as a feasibility study for an EHHA-wide haemoglobinopathy register, a centralized nurse counsellor service and an additional nurse counsellor over the period 2000–01 and 2001–02.

Another commendable and timely aim of the UK Forum on Haemoglobin Disorders is to facilitate collaborative research but it is vital that this must also involve user groups. Hogg (1999: 70) has pointed out that 'medical research tends to concentrate on narrow science-based questions that do not take account of the subjective views of users'. Another area of concern she highlights is that of securing informed consent and the conflict that can arise when the researcher is also the clinician. This is supported by a meeting on research into SCD and thalassaemia attended by over a hundred affected individuals, carers, relatives and professionals (Consumers for Ethics in Research 1995). Comments included 'I have been asked to join two research projects into thalassaemia. I felt that I was not given enough information, and that the doctors were putting pressure on me to join' (1995: 16) and 'I am worried because I was asked to join in a trial of hydroxyurea. I was reluctant but I felt I was being pressurised by my doctor

. . . We do want there to be more research, but we don't want to feel forced to take part in it' (1995: 15).

The UK Forum on Haemoglobin Disorders can also play a useful role in establishing the need for more accurate information concerning the estimated national prevalence of sickle cell disorders. The development of a national register for thalassaemia (Modell 1993) has provided useful data to chart the impact on approximately 800 affected individuals in Britain, including survival (Modell *et al.* 2000b) and there is a need for a similar register for SCD (Anionwu 1997). As it is estimated that there are over 10 times this number of individuals with SCD (Streetly *et al.* 1997) resources will be required for coordinating anonymized data from local or regional registers. Unsuccessful attempts to set up a register occurred between the late 1980s and early 1990s, following a donation for this purpose by the charity SCAR (Sickle Cell Anaemia Relief). Administrative difficulties and the suspicions of minority ethnic groups all seem to have contributed to this failure. In a letter responding to a paper on the low uptake for hydroxyurea within the UK (Olujohungbe *et al.* 1998), Davies and Roberts-Harewood (1998) described the setting up of a European register of patients with SCD treated with hydroxyurea. A more comprehensive European Haemoglobinopathy Registry (HER) has now been set up. It is to be hoped that those in charge of this new register will learn from the problems encountered in previous attempts to set them up.

The UK Forum has now demonstrated that it has the ability to become a political force to be reckoned with in a similar way to the model developed by those who have, for example, influenced that services for those with HIV/AIDS and cancer were identified as priorities for resources. If the UK Forum on Haemoglobin Disorders is to succeed it will need to establish greater involvement with user groups, and alliances with organizations facing similar issues and more sophisticated contacts with politicians.

We have already noted that another important success story in the development of haemoglobinopathy provision is the network of approximately 50 sickle cell and thalassaemia counselling centres employing a significant number of community based staff (also see Chapter 6). More recently, there has been the appointment of more specialist sickle cell and thalassaemia nurses within acute hospital settings (Anionwu 1996a). They are drawn from many diverse ethnic groups and are in an important position to contribute to the planning, delivery and audit of culturally sensitive services (Anionwu 1996a; Karretti 1997; Rochester-Peart 1997; Gould *et al.* 2000). More generally, localities employing such workers tend to offer better coordinated and better quality provision than areas that do not (Atkin *et al.* 1998a, 1998b). The Sickle and Thalassaemia Association of Counsellors (STAC), for example, initiated the successful UK-wide sickle cell and thalassaemia awareness weeks, held in July of each year. Building on the success of these specialist workers will be fundamental to any future improvements in sickle cell and thalassaemia services, although as we have noted earlier, the position of these workers is far from secure.

Another more specific development in the area – and another example of good practice – is an initiative led by Professor Bernadette Modell. The APoGI project, funded by the Wellcome Trust, provides detailed information on all the major haemoglobinopathies, including their carrier states. Information sheets can be printed from a CD-ROM or downloaded from the Internet by anybody involved in providing genetic counselling on haemoglobinopathies (such as GPs, midwives, haemoglobinopathy counsellors, paediatricians and haematologists). The information can also be accessed by other health and social care professionals as well as those from at-risk communities. Given that poor understanding among those providing support to those with haemoglobin disorders and their families is a major problem, the APoGi project is an important step forward in providing accessible information. (The web address is given at the end of this chapter.)

There are also important developments within the voluntary sector. Alliances of voluntary organizations such the Genetic Interest Group (GIG) – a national alliance of over 120 genetic charities that include some for sickle cell and thalassaemia disorders – could help bring coherence to sickle cell and thalassaemia provision. GIG's primary goal is 'to promote awareness and understanding of genetic disorders so that high quality services for people affected by genetic conditions are developed and made available to all who need them'. This organization provides opportunities to ensure that issues relating to sickle cell and thalassaemia do not become marginalized simply because they mainly affect minority ethnic communities. GIG has been instrumental in ensuring key agencies recognize the impact that this marginalization may have on the provision of services (Darr 1999).

Another important body that should not be allowed to ignore haemoglobinopathies is the Human Genetics Commission (HGC). Following a comprehensive review in May 1999, the UK government established the HGC as an advisory body to oversee how new developments in human genetics will impact on people and on NHS and health care. One of its key roles is to advise ministers on implications of the developments in human genetics and in particular to focus on social and ethical issues.

Conclusion

Those involved in the struggle to improve sickle cell and thalassaemia service provision since the mid-1970s have much to be proud of, particularly since their achievements have been made in the face of so much resistance, racism, ignorance and apathy. Alliances among voluntary and community groups and the enlightened commitment of some health and social care professionals and academics lie at the heart of this success. Their continuous pressure, for example, has forced the Department of Health to at least think about placing haemoglobinopathies on the mainstream NHS agenda. Such achievements should not be forgotten when recognizing, with justifiable concern, the huge number of issues that still need to be addressed to improve the quality of life for those affected by sickle cell or thalassaemia disorders. These include screening and genetic counselling services, comprehensive care within hospital and the community as well as the expansion of much needed research.

The future is open and neglect of haemoglobinopathies is not inevitable. Reminders of what has been accomplished will hopefully reinvigorate those activists who are somewhat tired and disillusioned at the difficulties they have experienced in this important arena of minority ethnic health. Strategy and struggle need to continue and ensure policy and practice developments adequately take account of haemoglobin disorders and meet the needs of at-risk populations, affected individuals and their families. This book, in its modest way, could helpfully inform these struggles by educating as well as motivating alliances with new and influential champions. As part of this, we have set out many of the outstanding gaps in health and social care provision as well as identified the potential opportunities that exist to rectify them. A critical understanding of these threats and opportunities are crucial in piloting a way forward and achieving a measurable improvement in the quality of sickle cell and thalassaemia services. Hopefully a book written in 10 years' time will present a very different and much more positive narrative that builds on the foundation of both present and previous struggles.

Appendix: Useful addresses and websites

UK Thalassaemia Society
19 The Broadway
Southgate Circus
London
N14 6PH
Tel: 020 8882 0011
www.ukts.org

Sickle Cell Society
54 Station Road
Harlesden
London
NW10 4UA
Tel: 020 8961 7795
www.sicklecellsociety.org

Organisation for Sickle Cell Anaemia Research (OSCAR)
Sickle Cell Community Centre
Tiverton Road
Tottenham
London
N15 6RT
Tel: 020 8802 3055

The National Co-ordinating Centre for Health Technology Assessment
Mailpoint 728
Boldrewood
University of Southampton
Southampton
SO16 7PX
www.ncchta.org

Mary Seacole Centre for Nursing Practice
Wolfson Institute of Health Sciences
Thames Valley University
Westel House
32–38 Uxbridge Road
Ealing
London W5 2BS
Tel: 020 8280 5109
www.maryseacole.com

APoGI Project: www.chime.ucl.ac.uk/APoGI/
APoGI (Accessible Publishing of Genetic Information) provides data on nearly all
haemoglobin disorders, including material on disorders and carrier states. It provides
an excellent source of information.

Black Information Link (BLINK): www.blink.org.uk
Black Information Link is a UK site for minority ethnic issues and includes informa-
tive pages on finance, business, legal matters, disability, education, Europe, human
rights and arts and culture. Its health information section has useful sickle cell links.

The Georgia Sickle Cell Information Centre: www.emory.edu/PEDS/SICKLE
This American website provides information for the sickle cell patient, their families
as well as welfare practitioners. It is an impressive site that covers both health and
social care issues.

Cooley's Anemia Foundation: www.thalassemia.org/home/net_op/h3.htm)
This is another American website providing extensive information on thalassaemia.
It is more medically orientated than the Georgia Sickle Cell site, but does include a
good introduction to the clinical consequences of thalassaemia disorders.

Human Genetics Commission: www.hgc.gov.uk
National Screening Committee: www.nsc.nhs.uk
Genetic Interest Group: www.gig.org.uk
Thalassaemia International Federation: www.thalassaemia.org.cy

Bibliography

Acheson, D. (1998) *Independent Inquiry into Inequalities in Health Report*. London: The Stationery Office.

Adams, J.G. 3rd (1994) Clinical laboratory diagnosis, in S.H. Embury, R.P. Hebbel, N. Mohandas and M.H. Steinberg (eds) *Sickle Cell Disease: Basic Principles and Clinical Practice*. New York: Raven Press.

Adams, R.J. (1994) Neurological complications, in S.H. Embury, R.P. Hebbel, N. Mohandas and M.H. Steinberg (eds) *Sickle Cell Disease: Basic Principles and Clinical Practice*. New York: Raven Press.

Adams, R.J., McKie, V.C., Hsu, L. *et al.* (1998) Prevention of a first stroke by transfusions in children with sickle cell anemia and abnormal results on transcranial Doppler ultrasonography, *New England Journal of Medicine*, 339(1): 5–11.

Advisory Committee on Genetic Testing (1997) *Code of Practice and Guidance on Human Genetic Testing Services Supplied Directly to the Public*. London: Department of Health.

Ahmad, W.I.U. (1993) Making black people sick: 'race', ideology and health research, in W.I.U. Ahmad (ed.) *'Race' and Health in Contemporary Britain*. Buckingham: Open University Press.

Ahmad, W.I.U. (1995) Reflections on consanguinity and birth outcome debate, *Journal of Public Health Medicine*, 16(4): 423–8.

Ahmad, W.I.U. (1996a) Family obligation and social change among Asian communities, in W.I.U. Ahmad and K. Atkin (eds) *'Race' and Community Care*. Buckingham: Open University Press.

Ahmad, W.I.U. (1996b) Consanguinity and related demons: science and racism in the debate on consanguinity and birth outcome, in C. Samson and N. South (eds) *Conflict and Consensus in Social Policy*. Basingstoke: BSA/Macmillan.

Ahmad, W.I.U. (2000) Introduction, in W.I.U. Ahmad (ed.) *Ethnicity, Disability and Chronic Illness*. Buckingham: Open University Press.

Ahmad, W.I.U. and Atkin, K. (1996a) *'Race' and Community Care*. Buckingham: Open University Press.

Ahmad, W.I.U. and Atkin, K. (1996b) Ethnicity and caring for a disabled child: the case of children with sickle cell or thalassaemia, *British Journal of Social Work*, 26: 755–75.

Ahmad, W.I.U. and Atkin, K. (2000) Primary care and haemoglobin disorders: a study of families and professionals, *Critical Public Health*, 10(1): 41–53.

Ahmad, W.I.U., Atkin, K. and Chamba, R. (2000) 'Causing havoc among their children'; parental and professional perspectives on consanguinity and childhood disability, in W.I.U. Ahmad (ed.) *Ethnicity, Disability and Chronic Illness*. Buckingham: Open University Press.

Ahmad, W.I.U., Baker, M.R. and Kernohan, E.E.M. (1991) General practitioners: perceptions of Asian and non-Asian patients, *Family Practice*, 8(1): 52–6.

Alexander, Z. (1999) *The Department of Health: Study of Black, Asian and Ethnic Minority Issues*. London: Department of Health.

ALG (2000) *Sick of being Excluded. Improving the Health and Care of London's Black and Minority Ethnic Communities*. London: Association of London Government.

Alleyne, J. and Thomas, V.J. (1994) The management of sickle cell crisis pain as experienced by patients and their carers, *Journal of Advanced Nursing*, 19: 725–32.

Alleyne, S.I., Wint, E. and Serjeant, G.R. (1977) Social effects of leg ulceration in sickle cell anaemia, *Southern Medical Journal*, 70: 213–14.

Allison, A.C. (1957) Properties of sickle-cell haemoglobin, *Biochemistry Journal*, 65: 212–19.

Angastiniotis, M.A. and Hadjimanas, M.G. (1981) Prevention of thalassaemia in Cyprus, *Lancet*, 1: 369–70.

Angastiniotis, M.A. and Modell, B. (1998) Global epidemiology of hemoglobin disorders, *Annals of the New York Academy of Sciences*, 850: 251–69.

Angastiniotis, M., Kyriakidou, S. and Hadjimanas, M. (1986) How thalassaemia was controlled in Cyprus, *World Health Forum*, 7: 291–7.

Anie, K., Smalling, B. and Fotopoulos, C. (2000) Group work: children and adolescents with sickle cell, *Community Practititoner*, 73(4): 556–8.

Anionwu, E.N. (1988) Health education and community development for sickle cell disorders in Brent. PhD thesis, Institute of Education: University of London.

Anionwu, E.N. (1989) Running a sickle cell centre: community counselling, in J.K. Cruickshank and D.G. Beever (eds) *Ethnic Factors in Health and Disease*. London: Wright.

Anionwu, E.N. (1992) Sickle cell disorders and the schoolchild, *Health Visitor*, 65(4): 120–2.

Anionwu, E.N. (1993) Sickle cell and thalassaemia: community experiences and official response, in W.I.U. Ahmad (ed.) *'Race' and Health in Contemporary Britain*. Buckingham: Open University Press.

Anionwu, E.N. (1996a) Sickle cell and thalassaemia: some priorities for nursing research, *Journal of Advanced Nursing*, 23(5): 853–6.

Anionwu, E.N. (1996b) Ethnic origin of sickle and thalassaemia counsellors: does it matter? in D. Kelleher and S. Hillier (eds) *Researching Cultural Differences*. London: Routledge.

Anionwu, E.N. (1997) District-based population registers for sickle cell disorders: a role for the haemoglobinopathy clinical nurse specialist? *Child Care, Health and Development*, 23(6): 431–5.

Anionwu, E.N. and Beattie, A. (1981) Learning to cope with sickle cell disease: a parent's experience, *Nursing Times*, 77: 1214–19.

Anionwu, E.N. and Jibril, H. (1986) *Sickle Cell Disease: A Guide for Families*. London: Longman.

Anionwu, E.N., Patel, N., Kanji, G., Renges, H. and Brozovic, M. (1988) Counselling for prenatal diagnosis of sickle cell disease and thalassaemia, *Journal of Medical Genetics*, 25: 769–72.

Anionwu, E.N., Walford, D., Brozovic, M. and Kirkwood, B. (1981) Sickle cell disease in a British urban community, *British Medical Journal*, 1: 283–6.

Anthias, F. (1992) *Ethnicity, Class, Gender and Migration*, Aldershot: Avebury.

Apperley, J.F. (1993) Bone marrow transplant for the haemoglobinopathies: past, present and future, *Clinical Haematolology*, 6: 299–325.

Ashiotis, T., Zachariadi, Z., Sofroniadou, K., Loukopoulos, D. and Stamatoyannopoulos, G. (1973) Thalassaemia in Cyprus, *British Medical Journal*, 2(857): 38–42.

Ashman, R. (1952) Are certain blood dyscrasias an effect of racial mixtures? *American Journal of Physical Anthropology*, 10: 217–18.

Associated Examining Board (1973) Human Biology. Paper 2. General Certificate of Education. Ordinary Level. Associated Examing Board. (43/2): 1–4.

Atkin, K. (1991) Health, illness, disability and black minorities: a speculative critique of present day discourse, *Disability, Handicap and Society*, 6(1): 37–47.

Atkin, K. (1992) Similarities and differences between carers, in J. Twigg (ed.) *Carers, Research and Practice*. London: HMSO.

Atkin, K. (1996) An opportunity for change: voluntary sector provision in a mixed economy of care, in W.I.U. Ahmad and K. Atkin (eds) *Race and Community Care*. Buckingham: Open University Press.

Atkin, K. and Ahmad, W.I.U. (1997) Genetic screening and haemoglobinopathies: ethics, politics and practice, *Social Science and Medicine*, 46(3): 445–58.

Atkin, K. and Ahmad, W.I.U. (2000a) Family care-giving and chronic illness: how parents cope with a child with a sickle cell disorder or thalassaemia, *Health and Social Care in the Community*, 8(1): 57–69.

Atkin, K. and Ahmad, W.I.U. (2000b) Living with a sickle cell disorder: how young people negotiate their care and treatment, in W.I.U. Ahmad (ed.) *Ethnicity, Disability and Chronic Illness*. Buckingham: Open University Press.

Atkin, K. and Ahmad, W.I.U. (2000c) Pumping iron: compliance with chelation therapy among young people who have thalassaemia major, *Sociology of Health and Illness*, 22(4): 500–24.

Atkin, K., Ahmad, W.I.U. and Anionwu, E.N. (1998a) Service support to families caring for a child with a sickle cell disorder or thalassaemia, *Health*, 2(3): 305–27.

Atkin, K., Ahmad, W.I.U. and Anionwu, E.N. (1998b) Screening and counselling for sickle cell disorders and thalassaemia: the experience of parents and health professionals, *Social Science and Medicine*, 47(11): 1639–51.

Atkin, K., Ahmad, W.I.U. and Anionwu, E.N. (2000) Service support to families caring for a child with a sickle cell disorder or beta thalassaemia major: parents' perspectives, in W.I.U. Ahmad (ed.) *Ethnicity, Disability and Chronic Illness*. Buckingham: Open University Press.

Atkin, K. and Rollings, J. (1993) *Community Care in a Multi-Racial Britain: A Critical Review of the Literature*. London: HMSO.

Atkin, K. and Rollings, J. (1996) Looking after their own? Family caregiving among Asian and Afro-Caribbean communities, in W.I.U. Ahmad and K. Atkin (eds) 'Race' and Community Care. Buckingham: Open University Press.

Bailey-Holgate, G. (1996) Educating young adults about sickle cell and thalassaemia, *Health Visitor*, 69(12): 499–500.

Bain, J. and Chapman, C. (1998) A survey of current United Kingdom practice for antenatal screening for inherited disorders of globin chain synthesis, *Journal of Clinical Pathology*, 51(5): 382–9.

Baker, M.S., Bandaranayake, R. and Schwieger, M.S. (1984) Differences in rate of immunization among ethnic groups, *British Medical Journal*, 288: 1075–8.

Baldwin, S. and Carlisle, J. (1994) *Social Support for Disabled Children and Their Families*. London: HMSO.

Balkaran, B., Char, G., Morris, J.S., Serjeant, B.E. and Serjeant, G.R. (1992) Stroke in a cohort of patients with homozygous sickle cell disease, *Journal of Paediatrics*, 120: 360–6.

Ballard, R. (1989) Social work with black people: What's the difference? in C. Rojeck, G. Peacock and S. Collins (eds) *The Haunt of Misery: Critical Essays in Social Work and Helping*. London: Routledge.

Ballas, S.K. (1990) Treatment of pain in adults with sickle cell disease, *American Journal of Haematology*, 34: 49–54.

Barbarin, O.A., Whitten, C.F. and Bonds, S.M. (1994) Estimated rates of psychological problems in urban and poor children with sickle cell anaemia, *Health and Social Work*, 19(2): 112–19.

Barnardo's (1993) *Report of Sickle Cell and Thalassaemia National Conference. The First Conference of the National Organisations*, Barnardo's Faith in the Black Country Community Project. Oldbury, West Midlands: Barnardo's.

Barrett-Connor, E. (1971) Bacterial infection and sickle cell anemia: an analysis of 250 infections in 106 patients and a review of the literature, *Medicine*, 50: 97–112.

Baughan, A.S.J. (1983) *Pain in Sickle Cell Disease: Proceedings of a Symposium Held at Central Middlesex Hospital*. London: Sickle Cell Society.

Bauman, Z. (1992) *Intimations of Postmodernity*. London: Routledge.

Baxter, C., Poonia, K., Ward, L. and Nadirshaw, Z. (1990) *Double Discrimination*. London: Kings Fund & Commission for Racial Equality.

Beattie, A. (1986) Community development for health: from practice to theory? *Radical Health Promotion*, 4: 279–84.

Beet, E.A. (1949) The genetics of sickle cell-trait in a Bantu tribe, *Annals of Eugenics (London)*, 14: 279–84.

Begum, N. (1994) Optimism, pessimism and care management: the impact of community care policies, in N. Begum, M. Hill and A. Stevens (eds) *Reflections: Views of Black Disabled People on Their Lives and Community Care*. London: CCETSW.

Beishon, S., Virdee, S. and Hagell, A. (1995) *Nursing in a Multi-Ethnic NHS*. London: Policy Studies Institute.

Benjamin, L.J., Dampier, C.D., Jacox, A. *et al.* (1999) *Guideline for the Management of Acute and Chronic Pain in Sickle-Cell Disease*. New York: American Pain Society.

Beratis, S. (1993) Psycho-social status in pre-adolescent children with beta thalassaemia, *Journal of Psychosomatic Research*, 37(3): 271.

Beresford, B. (1994) Resources and strategies: how parents cope with the care of a disabled child, *Journal of Child Psychology and Psychiatry*, 35(1): 171–209.

Beresford, B. (1996a) Coping with the care of a severely disabled child, *Health and Social Care in the Community*, 4(1): 30–40.

Beresford, B. (1996b) *Expert Opinions: A National Survey of Parents Caring for a Severely Disabled Child*. Bristol: Policy Press.

Beresford, B., Sloper, P., Baldwin, S. and Newman, T. (1996) *What Works in Services for Families with a Disabled Child?* Ilford, Essex: Barnardo's.

Beris, P., Darbellay, R. and Extermann, P. (1995) Prevention of α-thalassemia major and Hb Bart's hydrops fetalis syndrome, *Seminars in Hematology*, 32: 244–61.

Bessis, M. and Delpech, G. (1982) Sickle shape and structure: images and concepts 1840–1980, *Bloodcells*, 8: 359–435.

Bhakta, P., Katbamna, S. and Parker, G. (2000) South Asian experiences of primary health care teams, in W.I.U. Ahmad (ed.) *Ethnicity, Disability and Chronic Illness.* Buckingham: Open University Press.

Bhopal, R. and White, M. (1993) Health promotion for ethnic minorities, in W.I.U. Ahmad (ed.) *'Race' and Health in Contemporary Britain.* Buckingham: Open University Press.

Black, J. and Laws, S. (1986) *Living with Sickle Cell Disease: An Inquiry into the Need for Health and Social Service Provision for Sickle Cell Sufferers in Newham.* London: Sickle Cell Society.

Blakemore, K. and Boneham, M. (1995) *Age, Race and Ethnicity.* Buckingham: Open University Press.

Blakemore, K. and Drake, R. (1996) *Understanding Equal Opportunities Policies.* London: Harvester Wheatsheaf.

Blouin, M.J., Beauchemin, H., Wright, A. *et al.* (2000) Genetic correction of sickle cell disease: insights using transgenic mouse models, *Nature Medicine*, 6(2): 177–82.

Blum, R.W.M. (1992) Chronic illness and disability in adolescence, *Journal of Adolescent Health*, 13: 364–8.

Bodmer, W. and McKie, R. (1994) *The Book of Man: The Quest to Discover our Genetic Heritage.* London: Little, Brown & Co.

Borgna-Pignatti, C., Rugolotto, S., De Stefano, P. *et al.* (1998) *Annals of the New York Academy of Sciences*, 850: 227–31.

Bould, M. (1990) Asian carers: trapped within four walls, *Community Care*, 20 April (810): 17–19.

Bourdieu, P. (1977) *Outline of A Theory of Practice.* Cambridge: Cambridge University Press.

Bourdieu, P. (1984) *Distinction: A Social Critique of Taste.* London: Routledge.

Bowler, I. (1993) 'They're not the same as us?' midwives' stereotypes of South Asian maternity patients, *Sociology of Health and Illness*, 15(2): 157–78.

Bowman, J.E. and Murray, R.F. (1990) Genetic counselling and its adaptation to varying needs, in J.E. Bowman and R.F. Murray (eds) *Genetic Variation and Disorders in Peoples of African Origin.* Baltimore, MD: Johns Hopkins University Press.

Bradby, H. (1996) Genetics and racism, in T. Marteau and M. Richards (eds) *The Troubled Helix: Social and Psychological Implications of the New Human Genetics.* Cambridge: Cambridge University Press.

Braham, P., Rattansi, A. and Skellington, R. (1992) *Racism and Anti-Racism: Inequalities, Opportunities and Policies.* London: The Open University and Sage.

Brannen, J., Dodd, K., Oakley, A. and Storey, P. (1994) *Young People, Health and Family Life.* Buckingham: Open University Press.

British Committee for Standards in Haematology (1994) Guidelines for investigations of the alpha and beta thalassaemia traits, *Journal of Clinical Pathology*, 47: 289–95.

British Society for Haematology (1988) Guidelines for haemoglobinopathy screening, *Clinical Laboratory Haematology*, 10: 87–94.

Brock, D.J.H., Rodeck, C.H. and Ferguson-Smith, M.A. (1992) *Prenatal Diagnosis and Screening*. Edinburgh: Churchill Livingstone.

Broome, M. and Monroe, S. (1979) *Sickle Cell Anaemia: A Patient Perceived Assessment*. San Francisco, CA: Sickle Cell Anaemia Research and Education.

Brozovic, M. and Anionwu, E.N. (1984) Sickle cell disease in Britain, *Journal of Clinical Pathology*, 37: 1321–6.

Brozovic, M., Davies, S.C. and Brownell, A.I. (1987) Acute admissions of patients with sickle cell disease who live in Britain, *British Medical Journal*, 294: 1206–8.

Brozovic, M. and Stephens, A. (1991) *Guidelines for the Management of Sickle Cell Disease*. Geneva: WHO, Division of Noncommunicable Diseases & Health Technology. Hereditary Diseases Programme. (WHO/HDP/SCD/GL/91.2.)

Bury, M. (1991) The sociology of chronic illness, *Sociology of Health and Illness*, 13(4): 451–68.

Butt, J. (1994) *Same Service or Equal Service?* London: HMSO.

Cackovic, M., Chung, C., Bolton, L.L. and Kerstein, M.D. (1998) Leg ulceration in the sickle cell patient, *Journal of the American College of Surgeons*, 187(3): 307–9.

Cameron, E., Badger, F., Evers, H. and Atkin, K. (1989) Black old women, disability and health carers, in Jeffreys, M. (ed.) *Growing Old in the Twentieth Century*. London: Routledge.

Caminopetros, J. (1938) Recherches sur l'anemie erythroblastique infantile des peuples de la Mediterranean orientale, etude anthropologique, etiologique et pathogenique; la transmission hereditaire de la maladie, *Annals of Medicine*, 43: 104.

Cao, A., Gabutti, V., Modell, B. *et al.* (1992) *Management Protocol for the Treatment of Thalassaemia Patients*. New York: Cooley's Anemia Foundation of USA.

Cappellini, N., Cohen, A., Eleftherion, A. *et al.* (2000) *Guidelines for the Clinical Management of Thalassaemia*. Nicosia, Cyprus: Thalassaemia International Federation.

Carter, C.O. (1979) Recent advances in genetic counselling, *Nursing Times*, 75: 1795–8.

Cashmore, E. and Troyna, B. (1990) *Introduction to Race Relations*. London: The Falmer Press.

Castro, O. (1999) Management of sickle cell disease: recent advances and controversies, *British Journal of Haematology*, 107(1): 2–11.

Centre for Contemporary Cultural Studies (1982) *The Empire Strikes Back*. London: Hutchinson.

Chadwick, R. (1993) What counts as a success in genetic counselling? *Journal of Medical Ethics*, 19: 43–6.

Chamba, R., Ahmad, W.I.U. and Jones, L. (1998) *Improving Services for Asian Deaf People: Parents' and Professionals' Perspectives*. Bristol: Policy Press.

Chamba, R., Hirst, M., Lawton, D., Ahmad, W. and Beresford, B. (1999) *On the Edge: A National Survey of Minority Ethnic Parents Caring for a Severely Disabled Child*. Bristol: The Policy Press.

Chapple, J. and Anionwu, E.N. (1998) Health needs assessment: genetic services, in S. Rawaf and V. Bahl (eds) *Assessing the Health Needs of People from Ethnic Groups*. London: Royal College of Physicians.

Charache, S. and Davies, S.C. (1991) Teaching both the management and the molecular biology of sickle cell disease, *Academic Medicine*, 66(12): 48–9.

Charache, S., Terrin, M.L., Moore, R.D. *et al.* (1995) Effect of hydroxyurea on the frequency of painful crises in sickle cell anemia, *New England Journal of Medicine*, 332: 1317–22.

Chitty, L.S., Barnes, C.A. and Berry, C. (1996) Continuing with a pregnancy after a diagnosis of a lethal abnormality: experience of five couples and recommendations for management, *British Medical Journal*, 313(7055): 478–80.

Choiseul, M., May, A. and Jones, A. (1988) *Cardiff Sickle Cell and Thalassaemia Centre*. Cardiff: South Glamorgan Health Authority.

Clarfin, C.J. and Barbarin, O.A. (1991) Does 'telling' less protect more? Relationships among age, information disclosure and what children with cancer see and feel, *Journal of Pediatric Psychology*, 16: 169–82.

Clarke, A. (1991) Is non-directive counselling possible? *Lancet*, 338(8773): 998.

Clarke, A. and Parsons, B. (1997) *Culture, Kinship and Genes*. London: Macmillan Press.

Clarke, M. and Clayton, D. (1983) Quality of obstetric care provided for Asian immigrants in Leicestershire, *British Medical Journal*, 60: 866–79.

Cocking, I. and Athwal, S. (1990) A special case for treatment, *Social Work Today*, 21(22): 12–13.

Cohen, A.R. (1998) Sickle cell disease: new treatments, new questions (editorial), *New England Journal of Medicine*, 339: 42–4.

Collier, J. (1999) Tackling institutional racism, *British Medical Journal*, 318: 679.

Conley, C.L. (1980) Sickle cell anemia: the first molecular disease, in M.W. Wintrobe (ed.) *Blood, Pure and Eloquent*. New York: McGraw-Hill.

Conrad, P. and Bury, M. (1997) Anselm Strauss and the sociological study of chronic illness: a reflection and appreciation, *Sociology of Health and Illness*, 19 (3): 373–82.

Consumers for Ethics in Research (CERES) (1995) Special issue on sickle cell and thalassaemia, *Consumers for Ethics in Research*, 17 (Summer edition): 1–20.

Conyard, S., Krishnamurthy, M. and Dosik, H. (1980) Psychosocial aspects of sickle cell anaemia in adolescents, *Health and Social Work*, 5: 20–6.

Cook, J. and Meyer, J. (1915) Severe anemia with remarkable elongated and sickle-shaped red blood cells and chronic leg ulcer, *Archives of Internal Medicine*, 16: 644–51.

Cooley, T.B. and Lee, P. (1925) A series of cases of splenomegaly in children with anaemia and peculiar bone changes, *Transactions of the American Pediatric Society*, 37: 29.

Corker, M. and French, S. (1998) *Disability Discourse*. Buckingham: Open University Press.

Cowe, A. (1995) *Introduction to Haemophilia*. London: Haemophilia Society.

Cowen, L., Corey, M., Simmions, R. *et al.* (1984) Growing older with cystic fibrosis: psychological adjustment of patients more than sixteen years old, *Psychosomatic Medicine*, 46(4): 363–75.

Craig, G. and Rai, D.K. (1996) Social security and community care and 'race': the marginal dimension, in W.I.U. Ahmad and K. Atkin (eds) *'Race' and Community Care*. Buckingham: Open University Press.

Crawford, J. (1974) Sickle cell anaemia: action urged, *Race Today*, January: 8.

Crowley, J.P., Sheth, S., Capone, R.J. and Shilling, R.F. (1987) A paucity of thalassaemia trait in Italian men with myocardial infarction, *Acta Haematologica*, 78(4): 249–51.

Culley, L. (2000) Working with diversity: beyond the factfile, in C. Davies, L. Finlay and A. Bullman (eds) *Changing Practice in Health and Social Care*. Buckingham: Open University Press.

Currer, C. (1986) Concepts of mental well and ill-being: the case of Pathan mothers in Britain, in C. Currer and M. Stacey (eds) *Concepts of Health, Illness and Disease*. Leamington Spa: Berg.

Darr, A. (1990) The social implications of thalassaemia among Muslims of Pakistani origin in England – family experience and service delivery, PhD thesis, University College: University of London.

Darr, A. (1997) Consanguineous marriage and genetics – a positive relationship. A model for genetic health service delivery, in A. Clarke and E. Parsons (eds) *Culture, Kinship and Genes*. London: Macmillan Press.

Darr, A. (1999) *Access to Genetic Services by Minority Ethnic Populations. A Pilot Study*. London: Genetic Interest Group.

Darr, A. and Modell, B. (1988) The frequency of consanguineous marriage among British Pakistanis, *Journal of Medical Genetics*, 25: 186–90.

Davies, S., Modell, B. and Wonke, B. (1993) The haemoglobinopathies: impact upon black and ethnic minority people, in A. Hopkins and V. Bahl (eds) *Access to Health Care for People from Black and Ethnic Minorities*. London: Royal College of Physicians.

Davies, S.C. (1991) The vaso-occlusive crisis of sickle cell disease, *British Medical Journal*, 302: 1551–2.

Davies, S.C. (1994) Services for people with haemoglobinopathy, *British Medical Journal*, 308: 1051–2.

Davies, S.C., Cronin, E., Gill, M. *et al.* (2000) *Screening for Sickle Cell Disease and Thalassaemia: A Systematic Review with Supplementary Research*. Health Technology Assessessment Report 4(3).

Davies, S.C. and Oni, L. (1997) Management of patients with sickle cell disease, *British Medical Journal*, 315: 656–60.

Davies, S.C. and Roberts-Harwood, M. (1998) European register of patients with sickle cell disease treated with hydroxyurea is being set up, *British Medical Journal*, 317: 541.

Davies, S.C. and Wonke, B. (1991) The management of haemoglobinopathies, *Baillieres Clinical Haematology*, 4: 361–89.

Davis, J.K. and Wasserman, E. (1992) Behavioral aspects of asthma in children, *Clinical Pediatrics*, 31(1): 678–81.

Davis, L.R., Huehns, E.R. and White, J.M. (1981) Survey of sickle cell disease in England and Wales, *British Medical Journal*, 283: 1519–21.

de Montalembert, M., Girot, R., Mattlinger, B. and Lefrere, J.J. (1995) Transfusion-dependent thalassaemia: viral complications, *Seminars in Hematology*, 32: 280–7.

Deisseroth, A., Neinhuis, A., Lawrence, J. *et al.* (1978) Chromosomal localization of human beta globin gene on human chromosome 11 in somatic cell hybrids, *Proceedings of National Academy of Sciences (USA)*, 75: 1456–60.

Deisseroth, A., Neinhuis, A., Turner, P. *et al.* (1977) Localization of the human alpha-globin structural gene to chromosome 16 in somatic cell hybrids by molecular hybridization assay, *Cell*, 12: 205–18.

Department of Health (1993) *Report of a Working Party of the Standing Medical Advisory Committee on Sickle Cell, Thalassaemia and other Haemoglobinopathies*. London: HMSO.

Department of Health (1997) *The New NHS: Modern and Dependable*. London: The Stationery Office.

Department of Health (2000a) *The NHS Plan. A Plan for Investment. A Plan For Reform*. London: The Stationery Office.

Department of Health (2000b) *The Race Equality Agenda of the Department of Health: A Response to Ziggi Alexander's Study, The Department of Health: Study of Black, Asian and Ethnic Minority Issues*. London: Department of Health.

Department of Health/Social Services Inspectorate (1998) *'They Look After Their Own, Don't They?' Inspection of Community Care Services for Black and Ethnic Minority Older People*. London: Department of Health and Social Service Inspectorate.

Diggs, L.W., Ahmann, C.F. and Bibb, J. (1933) The incidence and significance of the sickle cell trait, *Journal of the American Medical Association*, 112: 695–701.

Dodge, J.A., Morrison, S., Lewis, P.A. *et al*. (1997) Incidence, population, and survival of cystic fibrosis in the UK, 1968–95, *Archives of Disease in Childhood*, 77(6): 493–6.

Dominelli, L. (1989) An uncaring profession? An examination of racism in social work, *New Community*, 15(3): 391–403.

Donahue, S.M., Wonke, B. and Hoffbrand, A.V. (1993) Alpha interferon in the treatment of chronic hepatitis C infection in thalassaemia major, *British Journal of Haematology*, 83: 491–7.

Dornbusch, S.M., Patersen, A.C. and Hetherington, E.M. (1991) Projecting the future of research on adolescence, *Journal of Research on Adolescence*, 1: 7–17.

Durrant, J. (1989) Moving forward in a multiracial society, *Community Care*, 792: iii–iv.

Dyson, S. (1997) Knowledge of sickle cell in a screened population, *Heath and Social Care in the Community*, 5(2): 84–93.

Dyson, S.M. (1998) Race, ethnicity and haemoglobin disorders, *Social Science and Medicine*, 47(1): 121–31.

Dyson, S. (1999) Genetic screening and ethnic minorities, *Critical Social Policy*, 19(2): 195–215.

Dyson, S., Davis, V. and Rahman, R. (1993) Thalassaemia: current community knowledge, *Health Visitor*, 66: 447–8.

Dyson, S., Davis, V. and Rahman, R. (1994) Thalassaemia: counselling and community education, *Health Visitor*, 67: 25–6.

Eaton, J.W. (1994) Malaria and the selection of the sickle gene, in S.H. Embury, R.P. Hebbel, N. Mohandas and M.H. Steinberg (eds) *Sickle Cell Disease: Basic Principles and Clinical Practice*. New York: Raven Press.

Ebata, A. and Moss, T. (1991) Coping and adjustment in distressed and healthy adolescents, *Journal of Applied Developmental Psychology*, 12: 33–54.

Eboh, W. and van den Akker, O. (1995) Service provision for sickle cell disease, *British Journal of Midwifery*, 3: 189–95.

Edelstein, S.J. (1986) *The Sickled Cell: From Myths to Molecules*. Cambridge, MA: Harvard University Press.

Edwards, S. (1993) A personal view of sickle pain, in J. Shankleman and A. May (eds) *Pain in Sickle Cell Disease: Setting Standards of Care*. (The proceedings of a one-day conference held on 19 September 1991, in the University of Wales College of Medicine, Cardiff, Wales on behalf of The Sickle and Thalassaemia Association of Counsellors). Cardiff: Community Health Unit, South Glamorgan Health Authority.

Eiser, C. (1990) *Chronic Childhood Disease: An Introduction to Psychological Theory and Research.* Cambridge: Cambridge University Press.

Eiser, C. (1994) Making sense of chronic disease. The eleventh Jack Tizard Memorial Lecture, *Journal of Child Psychology*, 35(8): 1373–89.

Elander, J. and Midence, K. (1996) A review of evidence about factors affecting quality of pain management in sickle cell disease, *The Clinical Journal of Pain*, 12: 180–93.

Embury, S.H., Hebbel, R.P., Mohandas, N. and Steinbery, M.H. (1994) *Sickle Cell Disease: Basic Principles and Clinical Practice.* New York: Raven Press.

Emery, D.W. and Stamatoyannopoulos, G. (1999) Stem cell gene therapy for the beta-chain hemoglobinopathies: problems and progress, *Annals of the New York Academy of Sciences*, 872: 94–107.

Emmel, V.E. (1917) A study of the erythrocytes in a case of severe anemia with elongated and sickle-shaped red blood corpuscles, *Archives of Internal Medicine*, 20: 586–98.

Evans, C. (1988) Children with sickle cell anaemia: parental relations, parent–child relations and child behaviour, *Social Work*, 33(2): 127–30.

Evans, J.A. and Hamerton, J.L. (1996) Limb defects and chorionic villus sampling, *Lancet*, 347: 484–5.

Falletta, J.M., Woods, G.M., Verter, J.I. *et al.* (1995) Discontinuing penicillin prophylaxis in children with sickle cell anaemia. Prophylactic penicillin study II, *Journal of Pediatrics*, 127: 685–90.

Farrah, M. (1986) Black elders in Leicester: an action research report on the needs of black elderly people of African descent from the Caribbean, *Social Services Research*, 1: 47–9.

Farrant, W. (1980) Stress after amniocentesis for high serum alpha-feto-protein concentrations, *British Medical Journal*, 281: 452.

Ferriman, A. (1984) Children die as 'sickle' screen plan is delayed, *Observer*, 11 March: 2.

Finch, J. and Mason, J. (1993) *Negotiating Family Responsibilities.* London: Routledge.

Finklestein, V. (1993) Disability: a social challenge or an administrative responsibility? in J. Swain, V. Finklestein, S. French and M. Oliver (eds) *Disabling Barriers – Enabling Environments.* London: Sage.

Firdous, R. and Bhopal, R.S. (1989) Reproductive health of Asian women: a comparative study with hospital and community perspectives, *Public Health*, 103: 307–15.

Fleming, A.F. (1982) *Sickle Cell Disease: A Handbook for the General Clinician.* Edinburgh: Churchill Livingstone.

Flynn, M. (1989) New right and social policy, *Policy and Practice*, 17(2): 97–102.

Flynn, R., Willams, G. and Pickard, S. (1996) *Markets and Networks: Contracting in Community Health Services.* Buckingham: Open University Press.

Fort, A.T., Morrison, J.C., Berreras, L., Diggs, L.W. and Fish, S.A. (1971) Counseling the patient with sickle cell disease about reproduction: pregnancy outcome does not justify the maternal risk! *American Journal of Obstetrics and Gynaecology*, 111: 324–7.

Foster, M.C. (1988) Health visitors' perspectives on working in multi-ethnic society, *Health Visitor*, 61: 275–8.

Foucault, M. (1977) *Discipline and Punish.* Harmondsworth: Penguin.

Fouche, H.H. and Switzer, P.K. (1949) Pregnancy with sickle cell anemia: review of the literature and report of cases, *American Journal of Obstetrics and Gynaecology*, 58: 468–77.

Fowler, M.G., White, J.K., Redding-Lallinger, R. *et al.* (1986) Neuropsychological deficits among school age children with sickle cell disease, *American Journal of Diseases of Childhood*, 140: 297–313.

France-Dawson, M. (1990) Sickle cell conditions and health knowledge, *Nursing Standard*, 4(35): 30–4.

France-Dawson, M. (1991) *Sickle Cell Conditions – The Continuing Need for Comprehensive Care Services: A Study of Patients' Views*. London: The Daphne Heald Research Unit, Royal College of Nursing.

Franklin, I.M. (1988) Services for sickle cell disease: unified approach needed, *British Medical Journal*, 296: 592.

Franklin, I. (1990) *Sickle Cell Disease: A Guide for Patients, Carers and Health Workers*. London: Faber and Faber.

Franklin, I. and Atkin, K. (1986) Employment of people with sickle cell disease and sickle cell trait, *Journal of the Society of Occupational Medicine*, 36(3): 76–9.

Frydenberg, E. (1997) *Adolescent Coping: Theoretical and Research Perspectives*. London: Routledge.

Fucharoen, S. and Winichagoon, P. (2000) Clinical and hematological aspects of hemoglobin E beta-thalassemia, *Current Opinion in Hematology*, 7(2): 106–12.

Fuggle, P., Shand, P.A.X., Gill, L.J. and Davies, S.C. (1996) Pain, quality of life and coping in sickle cell disease, *Archives of Disease in Childhood*, 75: 199–203.

Galacteros, F., Kleman, K., Caburi-Martin, J. *et al.* (1980) Cord blood screening for hemoglobin abnormalities by thin layer isoelectric focusing, *Blood*, 56: 1068–71.

Gaston, M.H., Verter, J.I., Woods, G. *et al.* (1986) Prophylaxis with oral penicillin in children with sickle cell anaemia: a randomized trial, *New England Journal of Medicine*, 314: 1593–9.

Geetz, C. (1983) *Local Knowledge: Further Essays in Interpretative Anthrology*. New York: Basic Books.

Geiss, S.K., Hobbs, S.A., Hammersley-Maercklein, G., Kramer, J.C. and Henley, M. (1992) Psychosocial factors related to perceived compliance with cystic fibrosis treatment, *Journal of Clinical Psychology*, 48(1): 99–103.

Gelpi, A.P. and Perrine, R.P. (1973) Sickle cell disease and trait in white populations, *Journal of the American Medical Association*, 244: 605–8.

Georganda, E.T. (1990) The impact of thalassaemia on body image, self-image, and self-esteem, *Annals of the New York Academy of Sciences*, 612: 466–72.

Gerrish, K., Husband, C. and Mackenzie, J. (1996) *Nursing for a Multi-Ethnic Society*. Buckingham: Open University Press.

Giardina, P.J. and Grady, R.W. (1995) Chelation therapy in β-thalassemia: the benefits and limitations of desferrioxamine, *Seminars in Hematology*, 32: 304–12.

Giddens, A. (1991) *Modernity and Self-Identity*. Cambridge: Polity Press.

Gil, K.M., Williams, D.A., Thompson, R.J. and Minney, T.R. (1991) Sickle cell disease in children and adolescents: the relations of child and parent pain coping strategies to adjustment, *Journal of Paediatric Psychology*, 16: 643–63.

Gill, F.M., Sleeper, L.A., Weiner, S.J. *et al.* (1995) Clinical events in the first decade in a cohort of infants with sickle cell disease, *Blood*, 86: 776–83.

Gill, P.S. and Modell, B. (1999) Thalassaemia in Britain: a tale of two communities, *British Medical Journal*, 317: 761–2.

Glader, B.E. and Look, K.A. (1996) Hematological disorders in children from Southeast Asia, *Paediatric Clinics of North America*, 43: 665–81.

Glasgow, D. (1980) *The Black Underclass*. New York: Jossey Bass.

Glendinning, C. (1985) *A Single Door*. London: Allen & Unwin.

Glendinning, F. and Pearson, M. (1988) *The Black and Ethnic Minority Elders in Britain: Health Needs and Access to Services*. Health Education Authority in Association with the Centre for Social Gerontology. Keele: University of Keele.

Globin Gene Disorder Working Party of the BCSH General Haematology Task Force (1994) Guidelines for the fetal diagnosis of globin gene disorders, *Journal of Clinical Pathology*, 47: 199–204.

Gould, D., Thomas, V. and Darlison, M. (2000) The role of the haemoglobinopathy nurse counsellor: an exploratory study, *Journal of Advanced Nursing*, 3(1): 157–64.

Graham, H. (1984) *Women, Health and the Family*. Brighton: Wheatsheaf.

Gramsci, A. (1957) *The Modern Prince and Other Writings*. London: Lawrence and Wishart.

Gray, A., Anionwu, E.N., Davies, S.C. and Brozovic, M. (1991) Patterns of mortality in sickle cell disease in United Kingdom, *Journal of Clinical Pathology*, 44: 459–63.

Green, J.M. (1992) Principles and practicalities of carrier screening: attitudes of recent parents, *Journal of Medical Genetics*, 29: 313–19.

Green, J. (1993) Ethics and late termination of pregnancy, *Lancet*, 342: 1179.

Green, J. and France-Dawson, M. (1997) Women's experiences of screening in pregnancy: ethnic differences in the West Midlands, in A. Clarke and B. Parsons (eds) *Culture, Kinship and Genes*. London: Macmillan Press.

Green, J.M. and Murton, F.E. (1996) Diagnosis of Duchenne muscular dystrophy: parents' experiences and satisfaction, *Child Care, Health and Development*, 22(2): 113–28.

Green, J. and Statham, H. (1996) Psychological aspects of prenatal screening and diagnosis, in T. Marteau and M. Richards (eds) *The Troubled Helix: Social and Psychological Implications of the New Human Genetics*. Cambridge: Cambridge University Press.

Hakim, L.S., Hashmat, A.I. and Macchia, R.J. (1994) Priapism, in S.H. Embury, R.P. Hebbel, N. Mohandas and M.H. Steinberg (eds) *Sickle Cell Disease: Basic Principles and Clinical Practice*. New York: Raven Press.

Hall, S., Bobrow, M. and Marteau, T.M. (2000) Psychological consequences for parents of false negative results on prenatal screening for Down's syndrome: retrospective interview study, *British Medical Journal*, 320: 407–12.

Hanson, C.L., Ciprang, J., Harris, M. *et al.* (1989) Coping styles in youths with insulin-dependent diabetes mellitus, *Journal of Consulting and Clinical Psychology*, 57: 644–51.

Harper, P. (1992) Genetics and public health, *British Medical Journal*, 304: 721.

Harper, P. (1998) *Practical Genetic Counselling*, 5th edn. Oxford: Butterworth Heinemann.

Harris, R., Lane, B., Harris, H. *et al.* (1999) National confidential enquiry into counselling for genetic disorders by non-geneticists: general recommendations and specific standards for improving care, *British Journal of Obstetrics and Gynaecology*, 106(7): 658–63.

Harrison, M. (1993) The black voluntary housing sector: pioneering pluralistic social policy in a difficult climate, *Critical Social Policy*, 13(3): 21–35.

Haynes, J.J., Manci, E. and Voelkel, N. (1994) Pulmonary complications, in S.H. Embury, R.P. Hebbel, N. Mohandas and M.H. Steinberg (eds) *Sickle Cell Disease: Basic Principles and Clinical Practice*. New York: Raven Press.

Headings, V.E. (1976) Association between type of health professional and judgements about prevention of sickling disorders, *Journal of Medical Education*, 51: 682–4.

Health Education Authority (1998) *Sickle Cell and Thalassaemia: Achieving Health Gain: Guidance for Commissioners and Providers*. London: HEA.

Held, D. (1989) *Political Theory and the Modern State*. Cambridge: Polity Press.

Heller, P., Best, W.R., Nelson, R.B. and Becktel, J. (1979) Clinical implications of sickle-cell trait and glucose-6-phosphate dehydrogenase deficiency in hospitalized black male patients, *New England Journal of Medicine*, 300: 1001–5.

Hellman, C.G. (2000) *Culture, Health and Illness*. Oxford: Butterworth Heinemann.

Herrick, J.B. (1910) Peculiar elongated and sickle shaped red blood corpuscles in a case of severe anemia, *Archives of Internal Medicine*, 6: 517–21.

Herzlich, C. (1973) *Health and Illness: A Social Psychological Analysis*. London: Academic Press.

Hickman, M., Modell, B., Greengross, C. *et al.* (1999) Mapping the prevalence of sickle cell and beta thalassaemia in England: estimating and validating ethnic-specific rates, *British Journal of Haematology*, 104: 860–7.

Hill, S.A. (1994) *Managing Sickle Cell Disease in Low Income Families*. Philadelphia, PA: Temple University Press.

Hillier, S. and Rahman, S. (1996) Childhood development and behavioural and emotional problems as perceived by Bangladeshi parents in East London, in D. Kelleher and S. Hillier (eds) *Researching Cultural Differences in Health*. London: Routledge.

Hilton, C., Osborne, M., Knight, S., Singhal, A. and Serjeant, G. (1997) Psychiatric complications of homozygous sickle cell disease among young adults in the Jamaican cohort study, *British Journal of Psychiatry*, 170: 69–76.

Hirst, M. and Baldwin, S. (1994) *Unequal Opportunities: Growing Up Disabled*. London: HMSO.

Ho, P., Hall, G.W., Luo, L.Y., Weatherall, D.J. and Thein, S.L. (1998) Beta-thalassaemia intermedia: is it possible consistently to predict phenotype from genotype? *British Journal of Haematology*, 100(1): 77–8.

Hodenpyl, E. (1898) A case of apparent absence of the spleen, with general compensatory lymphatic hyperplasia, *Medical Records*, 54: 695–8.

Hogg, C. (1999) *Patients, Power and Politics: From Patients to Citizens*. London: Sage.

Hoiberg, A., Ernst, J. and Uddin, D.E. (1981) Sickle cell trait and G-6-PD deficiency. Effects on health and military performance in black navy enlistees, *Archives of Internal Medicine*, 141: 1485–8.

Hopkins, A. and Bahl, V. (1993) *Access to Health Care for People from Black and Ethnic Minorities*. London: Royal College of Physicians.

Horton, J.A.B. (1874) *The Diseases of Tropical Climates and Their Treatment*. London: Churchill.

Howard, R.J. and Tuck, S.M. (1995) Sickle cell disease and pregnancy, *Current Obstetrics and Gynaecology*, 5: 36–40.

Howard, R.J., Lillis, C. and Tuck, S.M. (1993) Contraceptives, counselling and pregnancy in women with sickle cell disease, *British Medical Journal*, 306: 1735–7.

Howard, R.J., Tuck, S.M. and Pearson, T.C. (1995) Pregnancy in sickle-cell disease in the UK: results of a multicentre survey of the effect of a prophylactic blood transfusion on maternal and fetal outcome, *British Journal of Obstetrics and Gynaecology*, 102(12): 947–51.

Howrey, R.P., El-Alfondi, M., Phillips, K.L. *et al.* (2000) An in vitro system for efficiently evaluating gene therapy approaches to hemoglobinopathies, *Gene Therapy*, 7(3): 215–23.

Huck, J.G. (1923) Sickle cell anaemia, *Bulletin of Johns Hopkins Hospital*, 34: 335–44.

Hurtig, A.L. (1994) Relationships in families of children and adolescents with sickle cell disease, in K.B. Nash (ed.) *Psychosocial Aspects of Sickle Cell Disease: Past, Present and Future Directions of Research*. New York: The Haworth Press.

Hurtig, A.L. and Viera, C.T. (1986) *Sickle Cell Disease: Psychological and Psychosocial Issues*. Chicago, IL: University of Illinois.

Hurtig, A.L. and White, L.S. (1986) Psychosocial adjustment in children and adolescents with sickle cell disease, *Journal of Paediatric Psychology*, 11: 411–28.

Hutchinson, R.M. (1994) Umbilical cord blood banks for bone marrow transplantation in thalassaemia, *UK Thalassaemia News Review*, 60: 1–3.

Hyden, L.C. (1997) Illness and narrative, *Sociology of Health and Illness*, 19(1): 48–69.

Ingram, V.M. and Stretton, A.O.W. (1959) The genetic basis of the thalassaemia diseases, *Nature*, 184: 1903.

International Committee for Standardization for Haemoglobinopathies (1988) Recommendations for neonatal screening for haemoglobinopathies, *Clinical Laboratory Haematology*, 10: 335–45.

Jackson, D.E. (1972) Sickle cell disease: meeting a need, *Nursing Clinics of North America*, 7: 727–41.

Jain, C. (1985) *Attitudes of Pregnant Women to Antenatal Care*. Birmingham: West Midlands Health Authority.

Jani, B., Mistry, H., Patel, N., Anionwu, E.N. and Pembrey, M. (1992) A study of β thalassaemia in the Gujarati community of north London, *Paediatric Reviews and Communication*, 6: 191–2.

Jayaratnam, R. (1993) The need for cultural awareness, in A. Hopkins and V. Bahl (eds) *Access to Health Care for People from Black and Ethnic Minorities*. London: Royal College of Physicians.

Jenks, C. (1994) *Childhood*. London: Routledge.

Jensen, C.E. and Tuck, S.M. (1994) Endocrine problems in beta-thalassaemia major, *Contemporary Reviews in Obstetricians and Gynaecology*, 6: 133–6.

Jensen, C.E., Tuck, S.M. and Wonke, B. (1995) Fertility in β thalassaemia major: a report of 16 pregnancies, preconceptual evaluation and a review of the literature, *British Journal of Obstetrics and Gynaecology*, 102: 625–9.

Jess, M. (1989) Mum wins damages for sickle cell child, *The Voice*, 372: 1–3.

Jeyasingham, M. (1992) Acting for health: ethnic minorities and the community health movement, in W.I.U. Ahmad (ed.) *The Politics of 'Race' and Health*. Race Relations Research Unit, Bradford University.

Johnson, F.L., Look, A.T., Gockerman, J. *et al.* (1984) Bone marrow transplantation in a patient with sickle cell anemia, *New England Journal of Medicine*, 311: 780–3.

Johnson, S.B. (1988) Psychological aspects of childhood diabetes, *Journal of Child Psychology and Psychiatry*, 29: 729–38.

Journal of Medical Screening (1998) Screening brief. Antenatal screening for beta thalassaemia (and its variants), *Journal of Medical Screening*, 5: 215.

Kan, Y.W. and Dozy, A.M. (1978) Antenatal diagnosis of sickle cell anemia by DNA analysis of amniotic fluid cell, *Lancet*, 11: 910–12.

Kan, Y.W., Dozy, A.M., Alter, B.P., Frigoletto, F.D. and Nathan, D.G. (1972) Detection of the sickle gene in the human fetus: potential for intrauterine diagnosis of sickle-cell anemia, *New England Journal of Medicine*, 287: 1–5.

Kaplan, E., Zuelzer, W.W. and Neel, J.V. (1951) A new inherited abnormality of hemoglobin and its reactions with sickle cell hemoglobin, *Blood*, 6: 1240–59.

Kark, J.A., Posey, D.M., Schumacker, H.R. and Ruehle, C.J. (1987) Sickle cell trait as a risk factor for sudden death in physical training, *New England Journal of Medicine*, 317: 781–8.

Karretti, D. (1997) Antenatal counselling for the haemoglobinopathies, *Professional Care of the Mother and Child*, 7(2): 33–5.

Katbamna, S. (2000) *'Race' and Childbirth*. Buckingham: Open University Press.

Katbamna, S., Bhakta, P. and Parker, G. (2000) Perceptions of disability and care-giving relationships in South Asian communities, in W.I.U. Ahmad (ed.) *Ethnicity, Disability and Chronic Illness*. Buckingham: Open University Press.

Katbamna, S., Bhakta, P., Parker, G. and Ahmad, W.I.U. (1997) *The Needs of Asian Carers: A Selective Review of the Literature* (WP50 11/96). Leicester: Nuffield Community Care Studies Unit, University of Leicester.

Kelleher, D. and Hillier, S. (1996) *Researching Cultural Differences in Health*. London: Routledge.

Kelleher, D. and Islam, S. (1996) How should I live? Bangladeshi people and non-insulin-dependent diabetes, in D. Kelleher and S. Hillier (eds) *Researching Cultural Differences in Health*. London: Routledge.

Kelly, P., Kurtzberg, J., Vichinsky, E. and Lubin, B. (1997) Umbilical cord blood stem cells: application for the treatment of patients with hemoglobinopathies, *Journal of Paediatrics*, 130(5): 695–703.

Kevles, D.J. (1999) Eugenics and human rights, *British Medical Journal*, 319: 435–8.

Kinney, T.R., Helms, R.W., O'Branski, E.E., Ohene-Frempong, K. (1999) Safety of hydroxyurea in children with sickle cell anemia: results of the HUG-KIDS study, a phase 1/11 trial. Paediatric Hydroxyurea Group, *Blood*, 94(5): 1550–4.

Kleinman, A. (1988) *The Illness Narratives: Suffering, Healing and the Human Condition*. New York: Basic Books.

Kliewer, K. and Lewis, H. (1995) Family influences on coping processes in children and adolescents with sickle cell disease, *Journal of Paediatric Psychology*, 20(4): 511–25.

Koch, D.A., Giardina, P.J., Ryan, M., MacQueen, M. and Hilgartner, M.W. (1993) Behavioural contracting to improve adherence in patients with thalassaemia, *Journal of Paediatric Nursing*, 8(2): 106–11.

Kodish, E., Lantos, J., Stocking, C. *et al.* (1991) Bone marrow transplantation for sickle cell disease. A study of parents' decisions, *New England Journal of Medicine*, 325: 1349–53.

Konotey-Ahulu, F.I.D. (1968) Hereditary qualitative and quantitative erythrocyte defects in Ghana: an historical and geographical survey, *Ghana Medical Journal*, 7: 118–19.

Konotey-Ahulu, F.I.D. (1974) The sickle cell diseases, *Archives of Internal Medicine*, 133: 611–19.

Koshy, M. (1995) Sickle cell disease and pregnancy, *Blood Reviews*, 9: 157–64.

Koshy, M. and Burd, L. (1994) Obstetric and gynecologic issues, in S.H. Embury, R.P. Hebbel, N. Mohandas and M.H. Steinberg (eds) *Sickle Cell Disease: Basic Principles and Clinical Practice*. New York: Raven Press.

Kuliev, A.M. (1986) Thalassaemia can be prevented, *World Health Forum*, 7(3): 286–90.

Kumar, S., Powers, D., Allen, J. and Haywood, L. (1976) Anxiety, self concept and social adjustment in a clinic with sickle cell anaemia, *Journal of Paediatrics*, 88: 859–63.

Labropoulou, S. and Beratis, S. (1995) Psychosocial adjustment of thalassemia children's siblings, *Journal of Psychosomatic Research*, 39(7): 911–19.

Laird, L., Dezateux, C. and Anionwu, E.N. (1996) Neonatal screening for sickle cell disorder: what about the carrier infants? *British Medical Journal*, 313: 407–11.

Lakhani, N. (1999) Thalassaemia among Asians in Britain (letter), *British Medical Journal*, 318: 873.

Lambert, H. and Sevak, L. (1996) Is cultural difference a useful concept? Perceptions of health and sources of ill health among Londoners of South Asian origin, in D. Kelleher and S. Hillier (eds) *Researching Cultural Differences in Health*. London: Routledge.

Lancet (1983) Editorial: early infant death in sickle cell disease, *Lancet*, 1(8334): 1141–2.

Lancet (1999) Editorial: institutionalised racism in health care, *Lancet*, 353(9155): 765.

Law, I. (1996) *Racism, Ethnicity and Social Policy*. London: Harvester Wheatsheaf.

Lebby, R. (1846) Case of absence of the spleen, *Southern Journal of Medical Pharmacology*, 1: 481–3.

Lee, A., Thomas, P., Cupidore, L., Serjeant, B. and Serjeant, G.R. (1995) Improved survival in homozygous sickle cell disease: lessons from a cohort study, *British Medical Journal*, 311: 1600–2.

Lefrere, J.J., Girot, R. and European and Mediterranean WHO Working Group on Haemoglobinopathies (1989) Risk of HIV infection in polytransfused thalassemic patients [letter], *Lancet*, 2(8666): 813.

Leikin, S.L., Gallagher, D., Kinney, T.R. *et al.* (1989) Mortality in children and adolescents with sickle cell disease, *Paediatrics*, 84: 500–8.

Lemanek, K.L., Moore, S.L., Gresham, F.M., Williamson, D.A. and Kelley, M.L. (1986) Psychological adjustment of children with sickle cell anaemia, *Journal of Paediatric Psychology*, 11: 397–426.

LePontois, J. (1986) Adolescents with sickle cell anaemia: developmental issues, in A.L. Hurtig and C.T. Viera (eds) *Sickle Cell Disease: Psychological and Psychosocial Issues*. Urbana, IL: University of Illinois Press.

Letsky, E.A. (1976) A controlled trial of long-term chelation therapy in homozygous β-thalassaemia, in C.M. Peterson and J.H. Graziano (eds) *Iron Metabolism and Thalassaemia*. New York: Liss.

Levick, P. (1992) The Janus face of community care legislation: an opportunity for radical opportunities? *Critical Social Policy*, 12(1): 75–92.

Levitt, M. (2000) The gene shop at Manchester Airport, *New Genetics and Society*, 19(1): 77–87.

Lewis, J. and Meredith, B. (1988) *Daughters Who Care: Daughters Caring for Mothers at Home*. London: Routledge and Kegan Paul.

Liefner, R.J. and Vandenberghe, E.A. (1993) Sudden death in sickle cell disorders, *Journal of Royal Society of Medicine*, 86: 484–5.

Lipsky, M. (1980) *Street Level Bureaucracy: Dilemmas of the Individual in Public Service*. New York: Russell Sage.

Livingstone, F.B. (1985) *Frequencies of Haemoglobin Variants*. New York: Oxford University Press.

Loader, S., Sutera, C.J., Segelman, S.G., Kozyra, A. and Rowley, P.T. (1991) Prenatal hemoglobinopathy screening. IV: follow up of women at risk for a child with a clinically significant hemoglobinopathy, *American Journal of Medical Genetics*, 49: 1292–9.

Locker, D. (1997) Living with chronic illness, in G. Scamber (ed.) *Sociology as Applied to Medicine*. London: W.B. Saunders.

Logan, J. (2000) Haemoglobinopathy screening can be carried out in general practice (letter), *British Medical Journal*, 320: 1542.

Lorey, F., Cunningham, G., Shafer, F., Lubin, B. and Vichinsky, E. (1994) Universal screening for hemoglobinopathies using high-performance liquid chromatography: clinical results of 2.2 million screens, *European Journal of Human Genetics*, 2: 262–71.

Lucarelli, G., Giardini, C. and Baronciani, D. (1995) Bone marrow transplantation in thalassemia, *Seminars in Hematology*, 32: 297–303.

Lucarelli, G., Galimberti, M., Giardini, C. *et al.* (1998) Bone marrow transplantation in thalassemia. The experience of Pesaro, *Annals of the New York Academy of Sciences*, 850: 270–5.

Lunt, N. and Thornton, P. (1997) *Employment Policies for Disabled People*. London: Employment Department.

McIntyre, S. and Oldham, S. (1977) Coping with migraine, in C. Davies and M. Horobin (eds) *Medical Encounters*. London: Croom Helm.

Mack, A.K. (1989) Florida's experience with newborn screening, *Pediatrics*, 5: 861–3.

McKeown, T. (1979) *The Role of Medicine*. Oxford: Blackwell.

McKenzie, K. (1999) Something borrowed from the blues? We can use the Lawrence inquiry findings to eradicate racial discrimination in the NHS (editorial), *British Medical Journal*, 318: 616–17.

McKie, R. (1988) *The Genetic Jigsaw: The Story of the New Genetics*. Oxford: Oxford University Press.

Maclachlan, N.A. (1992) Amniocentesis, in D.J.H. Brock, C.H. Rodeck and M.A. Ferguson-Smith (eds) *Prenatal Diagnosis and Screening*. London: Churchill.

McNaught, A. (1987) *Health Action and Ethnic Minorities*. London: National Community Health Resource and Bedford Square Press.

Macpherson, W. (1999) *The Stephen Lawrence Inquiry: Implications for Racial Equality. Report of an Inquiry by Sir William Macpherson of Cluny* (CM 4262–1). London: The Stationery Office.

Madgwick, K.B. and Yardumian, A. (1999) A home blood transfusion service programme for β thalassaemia patients, *Transfusion Medicine*, 9: 135–8.

Mador, J.A. and Smith, D.H. (1989) The psychological adaptation of adolescences with cystic-fibrosis: the review of the literature, *Journal of Adolescent Health Care*, 10(2): 136–42.

Manchester Community Health Group for Ethnic Minorities (1981) *Sickle Cell Disease in Manchester: A Discussion Document for All Interested Groups and Particularly for Health Professionals*. Manchester: Manchester Community Health Council.

Mantadakis, E., Cavender, J.D., Rogers, Z.R., Ewalt, D.H. and Buchanan, G.R. (1999) Prevalence of priapism in children and adolescents with sickle cell anemia, *Journal of Pediatric Hematology/Oncology*, 21(6): 518–22.

Mao, X. (1998) Chinese geneticists' views of ethical issues in genetic testing and screening: evidence for eugenics in China, *American Journal of Human Genetics*, 63(3): 688–95.

Marteau, T.M. and Anionwu, E.N. (1996) Evaluating carrier testing: objectives and outcomes, in T. Marteau and M. Richards (eds) *The Troubled Helix: Social and Psychological Implications of the New Human Genetics*. Cambridge: Cambridge University Press.

Marteau, T. and Richards, M. (1996) *The Troubled Helix: Social and Psychological Implications of the New Human Genetics*. Cambridge: Cambridge University Press.

Marteau, T., Drake, H., Reid, M. *et al.* (1994) Counselling following diagnosis of fetal abnormality: a comparison between German, Portuguese and UK geneticists, *European Journal of Human Genetics*, 2(2): 96–102.

Marteau, T.M., Slack, J. and Kidd, J. (1992) Presenting a routine screening test in antenatal care: practice observed, *Public Health*, 106: 131–41.

Mason, V.R. (1922) Sickle cell anemia, *Journal of the American Medical Association*, 79: 1318–20.

Mavroudis, A. (1990) One day at a time, *UK Thalassaemia News Review*, 43: 4.

Maxwell, K. and Streetly, A. (1998) *Living with Sickle Pain*. London: Guys Department of Public Health Sciences, Kings and St Thomas' School of Medicine.

Maxwell, K., Streetly, A. and Bevan, D. (1999) Experiences of hospital care and treatment seeking for pain from sickle cell disease: qualitative study, *British Medical Journal*, 318: 1585–90.

May, A. and Choiseul, M. (1988) Sickle cell anaemia and thalassaemia: symptoms, treatment and effects on lifestyles, *Health Visitor*, 61: 212–14.

Mead, L. (1986) *Beyond Entitlement*. New York: Free Press.

Mentzer, W.C. (1994) Bone marrow transplantation, in S.H. Embury, R.P. Hebbel, N. Mohandas and M.H. Steinberg (eds) *Sickle Cell Disease: Basic Principles and Clinical Practice*. New York: Raven Press.

Michie, S., Bron, F., Bobrow, M. and Marteau, T.M. (1997) Non-directiveness in genetic counselling: an empirical study, *American Journal of Human Genetics*, 60: 40–7.

Michie, S. and Marteau, T. (1996) Genetic counselling: some issues of theory and practice, in T. Marteau and M. Richards (eds) *The Troubled Helix: Social and Psychological Implications of the New Human Genetics*. Cambridge: Cambridge University Press.

Midence, K. (1994) The effects of chronic illness on children, *Genetic Social and General Psychology Monographs*, 120(3): 311–26.

Midence, K. and Elander, J. (1994) *Sickle Cell Disease: A Psychological Approach*. Oxford: Radcliffe Medical Press.

Midence, K. and Elander, J. (1996) Adjustment and coping in adults with sickle cell disease: an assessment of research evidence, *British Journal of Health Psychology*, 1: 95–111.

Midence, K., McManus, C., Fuggle, P. and Davies, S. (1996) Psychological adjustment and family functioning in a group of British children with sickle cell disease: preliminary empirical findings and a meta-analysis, *British Journal of Clinical Psychology*, 35: 439–50.

Milner, P.F., Joe, C. and Burke, G.J. (1994) Bone and joint disease, in S.H. Embury, R.P. Hebbel, N. Mohandas and M.H. Steinberg (eds) *Sickle Cell Disease. Basic Principles and Clinical Practice*. New York: Raven Press.

Minuchin, P. (1974) Families and individual development: provocations from the field of family therapy, *Child Development*, 56: 289–302.

Modell, B. (1993) Concerted action on developing patient registers as a tool for improving service delivery for haemoglobin disorders, in G.N. Fracchia and M. Theophilatou (eds) *Health Services Research*, Amsterdam: IOS Press.

Modell, B. and Anionwu, E.N. (1996) Guidelines for screening for haemoglobin disorders: service specifications for low and high prevalence DHAs, in *Ethnicity and Health: Reviews of Literature and Guidance for Purchasers in the Areas of Cardiovascular Disease, Mental Health and Haemoglobinopathies.* (CRD Report No 5.) York: University of York NHS Centres for Reviews and Dissemination and Social Policy Research Unit.

Modell, B. and Berdoukas, V. (1984) *The Clinical Approach to Thalassaemia.* London: Grune and Stratton.

Modell, B., Harris, R., Lane, B. *et al.* (2000a) Informed choice in genetic screening for thalassaemia during pregnancy: audit from a national confidential inquiry, *British Medical Journal*, 320: 337–40.

Modell, B., Khan, M. and Darlison, M. (2000b) Survival in beta thalassaemia major in the United Kingdom: data from the UK thalassaemia register, *Lancet*, 355(9220): 2051–2.

Modell, B. and Kuliev, A.M. (1991) Services for thalassaemia as a model for cost-benefit analysis of genetics services, *Journal of Inherited Metabolic Disease*, 14(4): 640–51.

Modell, B., Kuliev, A.M. and Wagner, M. (1991) *Community Genetics Services in Europe.* Copenhagen: WHO Regional Publications.

Modell, B. and Kuliev, A.M. (1992) *Social and Genetic Implications of Customary Consanguineous Marriage Among British Pakistanis.* London: The Galton Institute.

Modell, B., Letsky, E.A., Flynn, D.M., Peto, R. and Weatherall, D.J. (1982) Survival and desferrioxamine in thalassaemia major, *British Medical Journal*, 284: 1081–4.

Modell, M., Wonke, B., Anionwu, E.N. *et al.* (1998) A multidisciplinary approach for improving services in primary care: a randomised trial of screening for haemoglobin disorders, *British Medical Journal*, 317: 788–91.

Modood, T., Bieshson, S. and Virdee, S. (1994) *Changing Ethnic Identities.* London: Policy Studies Institute.

Modood, T., Berthould, R., Lakey, J. *et al.* (1997) *Ethnic Minorities in Britain: Diversity and Disadvantage.* London: Policy Studies Institute.

Molock, S.D. and Belgrave, F.Z. (1994) Depression and anxiety in patients with sickle cell disease: conceptual and methodological considerations, in K.B. Nash (ed.) *Psychosocial Aspects of Sickle Cell Disease: Past, Present and Future Directions of Research.* New York: The Haworth Press.

Moncrieff, A. and Whitbey, E.H. (1934) Cooley's anaemia, *Lancet*, ii: 648.

Moore, M., Beazley, S. and Maelzer, J. (1997) *Researching Disability Issues.* Buckingham: Open University Press.

Morris, J. (1991) *Pride Against Prejudice; Transforming Attitudes to Disability.* London: Women's Press.

Morris, J. (1998) *Still Missing?* London: Trust.

Mozzi, F., Rebulla, P. and Lillo, F. (1992) HIV and HTLV-1 infection in 1,305 transfusion-dependent thalassemics in Italy, *AIDS*, 6: 505–8.

Mukerji, M. (1938) Cooley's anaemia (erythroblastic or Mediterranean anaemia), *Indian Journal of Paediatrics*, 5: 1–7.

Murray, J., Cuckle, H.S., Taylor, G. and Hewison, J. (1997) Screening for fragile X syndrome, Health Technology Assessment Report, 1(4).

Murray, J., Cuckle, H.S., Taylor, G., Littlewood, J. and Hewison, J. (1999) Screening for cystic fibrosis, Health Technology Assessment Report, 3(8).

Murray, N. and May, A. (1988) Painful crises in sickle cell disease: patients' perspectives, *British Medical Journal*, 297: 452–4.

Nagel, R.L. (1994) Origins and dispersion of the sickle gene, in S.H. Embury, R.P. Hebbel, N. Mohandas and M.H. Steinberg (eds) *Sickle Cell Disease: Basic Principles and Clinical Practice*. New York: Raven Press.

Nash, K.B. (1977) Family counseling in sickle cell anemia, *Urban Health*, 44–7.

Nash, K.B. (1990) Growing up with thalassemia: a chronic disorder, *Annals of the New York Academy of Sciences*, 612: 442–50.

Nash, K.B. (1994) *Psychosocial Aspects of Sickle Cell Disease: Past, Present and Future Directions of Research*. New York: The Haworth Press.

Nathan, D.G. and Weatherall, D.J. (1999) Academia and industry: lessons from the unfortunate events in Toronto, *Lancet*, 353(9155): 771–2.

National Health Service Executive (1998) *Tackling Racial Harassment in the NHS: A Plan for Action*. London: Department of Health.

National Health Service Executive (2000) *The Vital Connection: An Equalities Framework for the NHS*. London: Department of Health.

National Health Service Management Executive (1994) *Sickle Cell Anaemia*. London: Department of Health.

Neel, J.V. (1947) The clinical detection of the genetic carriers of inherited disease, *Medicine*, 26: 115–53.

Neel, J.V. (1949) The inheritance of sickle cell anaemia, *Science*, 110: 64–6.

Neel, J.V., Kaplan, E. and Zuelzer, W.W. (1953) Further studies on hemoglobin C. I. A description of three additional families segregating for hemoglobin C and sickle cell hemoglobin, *Blood*, 8: 724–34.

Nettles, A.L. (1994) Scholastic performance of children with sickle cell disease, in K.B. Nash (ed.) *Psychosocial Aspects of Sickle Cell Disease: Past, Present and Future Directions of Research*. New York: The Haworth Press.

Noll, R.B., Yousa, L.A., Vannatta, K. *et al.* (1995) Social competence of children with sickle cell anaemia, *Journal of Paediatric Psychology*, 20(2): 165–72.

Noller, P. and Callan, V.J. (1991) *Adolescences in the Family*. New York: Routledge.

Nuffield Council on Bioethics (1993) *Genetic Screening: Ethical Issues*. London: Nuffield Council on Bioethics.

Office of Public Management (1996) *Responding to Diversity: A Study of Commissioning Issues and Good Practice in Purchasing Minority*. London: Office of Public Management.

Old, J. (1996) Haemoglobinopathies, *Prenatal Diagnosis*, 16: 1181–6.

Old, J., Fitches, A., Heath, C. *et al.* (1986) First trimester fetal diagnosis for the haemoglobinopathies: report on 200 cases, *Lancet*, ii: 763–8.

Old, J., Ward, R.H.T., Petrou, M. *et al.* (1982) First trimester fetal diagnosis for haemoglobinopathies: three cases, *Lancet*, 2: 1413–16.

Oliver, M. (1996) *Understanding Disability from Theory to Practice*. Basingstoke: Macmillan.

Olivieri, N.F. (1996) Long-term therapy with deferiprone, *Acta Haematology*, 95: 37–48.

Olivieri, N.F., Nathan, D.G. and MacMillan, J.H. (1994) Survival in medically treated patients with homozygous beta thalassemia, *New England Journal of Medicine*, 331: 574–8.

Olujohungbe, A., Cinkotai, K.I. and Yardumian, A. (1998) Hydroxyurea therapy for sickle cell disease in Britain: disappointing recruitment despite promising results, *British Medical Journal*, 316: 1689–90.

O'Neale, V. (2000) *Excellence Not Excuses: Inspection of Services for Ethnic Minority Children and Families.* London: Department of Health.

Orsini, A. and Boyer, G. (1961) *La talassemia a Marsiglia; dati sulla frequenza ed osservazioni su alcuni aspetti clinici, terapeutici ed assistenziali. Il problema sociale della microcitemia e del morbo di Cooley.* Rome, Italy.

Ostrowsky, J.T., Lippman, A. and Scriver, C.R. (1985) Cost–benefit analysis of a thalassaemia disease prevention program, *American Journal of Public Health*, 75(7): 732–6.

Owen, D. (1994) *Ethnic Minorities in Britain.* Coventry: Centre for Research in Ethnic Relation, University of Warwick.

Pediatrics (1989) Newborn screening for sickle cell disease and other hemoglobinopathies, *Paediatrics Supplement*, 83(5): 813–914.

Pallister, C.J. (1992) Thalassaemia: a preventable disease? *Professional Nurse*, 666–9.

Parker, G. (1990) *With Due Care and Attention: A Review of Research on Informal Care*, 2nd edn. London: Family Policy Studies Centre.

Parker, G. (1993) A four way stretch? The politics of disability and caring, in J. Swain, V. Finkelstein, S. French and M. Oliver (eds) *Disabling Barriers – Enabling Environments.* London: Sage.

Parsons, L., McFarlane, A. and Golding, J. (1993) Pregnancy, birth and maternity care, in W.I.U. Ahmad (ed.) *'Race' and Health in Contemporary Britain.* Buckingham: Open University Press.

Parsons, E. and Atkinson, P. (1992) Genetic risk and reproduction, *Sociological Review*, 41(4): 679–706.

Pauling, L., Itano, H.A., Singer, S.J. and Wells, I.C. (1949) Sickle cell anaemia, a molecular disease, *Science*, 110: 543–8.

Pembrey, M.E. and Anionwu, E.N. (1996) Ethical aspects of genetic diagnosis and screening, in D.L. Rimoin, J.M. Connor, R.E. Pyeritz and A.E.H. Emery (eds) *Principles and Practice of Medical Genetics*, 3rd edn. Edinburgh: Churchill Livingstone.

Pembrey, M.E., Barnicoat, A.J., Carmichael, B., Bobrow, M. and Turner, G. (2001) An assessment of screening strategies for fragile X syndrome in the UK, *Health Technology Assessment*, 5(7).

Penna, A. and O'Brien, M. (1996) Postmodernism and social policy: a small step forwards? *Journal of Social Policy*, 25(1): 39–62.

Petrou, M. and Modell, B. (1995) Prenatal screening for haemoglobin disorders, *Prenatal Diagnosis*, 15(13): 1275–95.

Petrou, M., Brugiatelli, M., Old, J. (1992a) Alpha thalassaemia hydrops fetalis in the UK: the importance of screening pregnant women of Chinese, other South East Asian and Mediterranean extraction for alpha thalassaemia trait, *British Journal of Obstetrics and Gynaecology*, 99: 985–9.

Petrou, M., Brugiatelli, M., Ward, R.H.T. and Modell, B. (1992b) Factors affecting the uptake of prenatal diagnosis for sickle cell disease, *Journal of Medical Genetics*, 29: 820–3.

Petrou, M., Modell, B., Darr, A. *et al.* (1990) Antenatal diagnosis: how to deliver a comprehensive service in the United Kingdom, *Annals of the New York Academy of Sciences*, 612: 251–63.

Petrou, M., Ward, R.H.T., Modell, B. *et al.* (1983) Obstetric outcome in first trimester fetal diagnosis for the haemoglobinopathies, *Lancet*, 2: 1251.

Phelps, S.B. and Jarvis, P.A. (1994) Coping in adolescence: empirical evidence for a theoretically based approach to assessing coping, *Journal of Youth and Adolescence*, 23(3): 359–71.

Pinder, C. (1985) *Community Start Up*. Cambridge: National Extension College/ National Federation of Community Organisations.

Piomelli, S. (1995) The management of patients with Cooley's anemia: transfusions and splenectomy, *Seminars in Hematology*, 32: 262–8.

Plant, R., Lesser, H. and Taylor-Gooby, P. (1989) *Political Philosophy and Social Welfare Essays on the Normative*. London: Routledge.

Platt, O.S., Brambilla, D.J., Rosse, W.F. *et al.* (1994) Mortality in sickle cell disease – life expectancy and risk factors for early death, *New England Journal of Medicine*, 330: 1639–43.

Politis, C., Di Palma, A., Fisfis, M. *et al.* (1990) Social integration of the older thalassaemic patient, *Archives of Disease in Childhood*, 65: 984–6.

Politis, C., Richardson, C. and Yantopoulos, J.G. (1991) Public knowledge of thalassaemia in Greece and current concepts of the social-status of the thalassemic patient, *Social Science and Medicine*, 32(1): 59–64.

Potrykus, C. (1991) Sickle cell: call for better services and universal screening, *Health Visitor*, 64(12): 404–5.

Potrykus, C. (1993) Sickle cell: black counsellors under pressure, *Health Visitor*, 6(7): 239–41.

Powars, D.R. (1975) Natural history of sickle cell disease – the first ten years, *Seminars in Hematology*, 12: 267–85.

Powars, D.R. (1994a) Sickle cell disease in non-black persons, *Journal of the American Medical Association*, 271(23): 1885.

Powars, D.R. (1994b) Natural history of disease: the first two decades, in S.H. Embury, R.P. Hebbel, N. Mohandas and M.H. Steinberg (eds) *Sickle Cell Disease: Basic Principles and Clinical Practice*. New York: Raven Press.

Powars, D.R., Elliott-Mills, D.D., Chane, L. *et al.* (1991) Chronic renal failure in sickle cell disease: risk factors, clinical course, and mortality, *Annals of Internal Medicine*, 115(8): 614–20.

Powars, D.R., Overturf, G., Weiss, J., Lee, S. and Chan, L. (1981) Pneumococcal septicemia in children with sickle cell anemia: changing trend of survival, *Journal of the American Medical Association*, 245: 1839–42.

Powell, W.N., Rodarte, J.G. and Neel, J.V. (1950) The occurrence in a family of Sicilian ancestry of the traits for both sickling and thalassemia, *Blood*, 5: 887–97.

Prashar, U., Anionwu, E.N. and Brozovic, M. (1985) *Sickle Cell Anaemia: Who Cares?* London: Runnymede Trust.

Propper, R.D., Cooper, B. and Rufo, R.R. (1977) Continuous subcutaneous administration of desferrioxamine in patients with iron overload, *New England Journal of Medicine*, 297: 418–23.

Quine, L. and Pahl, J. (1985) Examining the causes of stress in families with severely mentally handicapped children, *British Journal of Social Work*, 15: 501–17.

Quinn, C.T. and Buchanan, G.R. (1999) The acute chest syndrome of sickle cell disease, *Paediatrics*, 135(4): 416–22.

Ranney, H.M. (1994) Historical milestones, in S.H. Embury, R.P. Hebbel, N. Mohandas and M.H. Steinberg (eds) *Sickle Cell Disease: Basic Principles and Clinical Practice*. New York: Raven Press.

Rapp, R. (1988) Chromosomes and communication: the discourse of genetic counselling, *Medical Anthropology Quarterly*, 2(2): 143–57.

Ratip, S. and Modell, B. (1996) Psychological and sociological aspects of the thalassemias, *Seminars in Haematology*, 33(1): 53–65.

Ratip, S., Skuse, D., Porter, J. *et al.* (1995) Psychosocial and clinical burden of thalassaemia intermedia and its implications for prenatal diagnosis, *Archives of Disease in Childhood*, 72: 408–12.

Rawaf, S. and Bahl, V. (1998) *Assessing Health Needs of People from Minority Ethnic Groups*. London: Royal College of Physicians.

Rebulla, P., Mozzi, F., Coutinho, G., Locatelli, E. and Sirchia, G. (1992) Antibody to hepatitis C virus in 1,305 Italian multiply transfused thalassaemics: a comparison of first and second generation tests (letter), *Transfusion Medicine*, 2: 69–70.

Reilly, P.R. (1992) Medicolegal aspects: USA, in D.J.H. Brock, C.H. Rodeck and M.A. Ferguson-Smith (eds) *Prenatal Diagnosis and Screening*. Edinburgh: Churchill Livingstone.

Richards, M. (1993) The new genetics: some issues for social scientists, *Sociology of Health and Illness*, 15(5): 567–86.

Richards, M.P.M. and Green, J.M. (1993) Attitudes toward prenatal screening for fetal abnormality and detection of carriers of genetic disease: a discussion paper, *Journal of Reproductive and Infant Psychology*, 11: 49–56.

Roberts, I.A.G. (1994) Bone marrow transplantation in sickle cell anaemia, *Journal of Internal Medicine*, 236: 483–6.

Rocherson, Y. (1988) The Asian mother and baby campaign: the construction of ethnic minorities' health needs, *Critical Social Policy*, 22: 4–23.

Rochester-Peart, C. (1997) Specialist nurse support for clients with blood disorders, *Nursing Times*, 93(41): 52–3.

Rodgers, G.P. and Rachmilewitz, E.A. (1995) Novel treatment options in the severe beta-globin disorders, *British Journal of Haematology*, 91: 263–8.

Rogers, D.W., Clarke, J.M., Cupidore, L. *et al.* (1978) Early deaths in Jamaican children with sickle cell disease, *British Medical Journal*, 1: 1515–16.

Rothman, B.K. (1988) *The Tentative Pregnancy: Prenatal Diagnosis and the Future of Motherhood*. London: Pandora.

Rothman, B.K. (1993) *The Tentative Pregnancy: How Amniocentesis Changes the Experience of Pregnancy*. New York: Norton.

Roulstone, A. (1998) *Enabling Technology: Disabled People, Work and New Technology*. Buckingham: Open University Press.

Rowley, P.T. (1989) Parental receptivity to neonatal sickle cell trait identification, *Paediatrics*, 63: 891–3.

Royal College of Physicians (1989) *Prenatal Diagnosis and Genetic Screening: Community and Service Implications*. London: Royal College of Physicians.

Sadelain, M. (1997) Genetic treatment of the hemoglobinopathies: recombinations and new combinations, *British Journal of Haematology*, 98(2): 247–53.

Samperi, D., Mancuso, G.R., Dibenedetto, S.P. *et al.* (1991) High performance liquid chromatography (HPLC): a simple method to quantify Hb C, O-Arab, Agenogi and F, *Clinical Laboratory Haematology*, 13: 169–75.

Sashidaran, S.P. and Francis, E. (1993) Epidemiology, ethnicity and schizophrenia, in W.I.U. Ahmad (ed.) *'Race' and Health in Contemporary Britain*. Buckingham: Open University Press.

Savitt, T.L. and Goldberg, M.F. (1989) Herrick's 1910 case report of sickle anemia: the rest of the story, *Journal of the American Medical Association*, 261: 266–71.

Sawyer, S.M., Rosier, M.J., Phelan, P.D. and Bowes, G. (1995) The self-image of adolescents with cystic fibrosis, *Journal of Adolescent Health*, 16: 204–8.

Scambler, G. (1987) *Sociological Theory and Medical Sociology*. Tavistock: London.

Scambler, G. (1996) *Sociology as Applied to Medicine*. London: W.B. Saunders.

Science and Technology Committee of the House of Commons (1995) *Human Genetics: The Science And Its Consequences (Volume 1: Report and Minutes of Proceedings)*. London: HMSO.

Sears, D.A. (1994) Sickle cell trait, in S.H. Embury, R.P. Hebbel, N. Mohandas and M.H. Steinberg (eds) *Sickle Cell Disease: Basic Principles and Clinical Practice*. New York: Raven Press.

Serjeant, G.R. (1992) *Sickle Cell Disease*, 2nd edn. Oxford: Oxford University Press.

Serjeant, G.R. (1997) Sickle-cell disease, *Lancet*, 350: 725–30.

Shakespeare, T. (1999) Losing the plot? Medical and activist discourses of contemporary genetics and disability, *Sociology of Health and Illness*, 21(5): 669–88.

Shankleman, J. and May, A. (1993) *Pain in Sickle Cell Disease: Setting Standards of Care*. (The proceedings of a one-day conference held on 19 September 1991 at the University of Wales College of Medicine, Cardiff, on behalf of The Sickle and Thalassaemia Association of Counsellors.) Cardiff: Community Health Unit, South Glamorgan Health Authority.

Shapiro, B.S. and Ballas, S.K. (1994) The acute painful episode, in S.H. Embury, R.P. Hebbel, N. Mohandas and M.H. Steinberg (eds) *Sickle Cell Disease: Basic Principles and Clinical Practice*. New York: Raven Press.

Shapiro, B.S., Dinges, D.F., Orne, E.C. *et al.* (1995) Home management of sickle-related pain in children and adolescents: natural history and impact on school attendance, *Pain*, 61: 139–44.

Shickle, D. and May, A. (1989) Knowledge and perceptions of haemoglobinopathy carrier screening among general practitioners in Cardiff, *Journal of Medical Genetics*, 26: 109–12.

Shiloh, S. (1996) Decision making in the context of genetic risk, in T. Marteau and M. Richards (eds) *The Troubled Helix: Social and Psychological Implications of the New Human Genetics*. Cambridge: Cambridge University Press.

Sickle Cell Disease Guideline Panel (1993) *Sickle Cell Disease: Screening, Diagnosis, Management, and Counseling in Newborns and Infants: Clinical Practice Guideline (Number 6)*. Rockville, MD: U.S. Department of Health and Human Services.

Sickle Cell Society (1981) *Sickle Cell Disease: The Need for Improved Services*. London: Sickle Cell Society.

Sickle Cell Society (2000) *Sickle Cell News Review: Millennium Issue*. London: Sickle Cell Society.

Silverman, N.S. and Wapner, R.J. (1992) Chorionic villus sampling, in D.J.H. Brock, C.H. Rodeck and M.A. Ferguson-Smith (eds) *Prenatal Diagnosis and Screening*. London: Churchill.

Silvestroni, E. and Bianco, I. (1952) Genetic aspects of sickle cell anemia and microdrepanocytic disease, *Blood*, 7: 429–35.

Sinnema, G. (1992) Youths with chronic illness and disability on their way to social and economic participation: a health care perspective, *Journal of Adolescent Health*, 13: 369–71.

Skellington, R. (1992) *'Race' in Britain Today*. London: Sage.

Sloper, P. (1996) Needs and responses of parents following the diagnosis of childhood cancer, *Child: Care, Health and Development*, 22: 187–202.

Sloper, P. and Turner, S. (1992) Service needs of families of children with severe physical disability, *Child: Care, Health and Development*, 18: 259–82.

Sloper, P. and Turner, S. (1993a) Determinants of parental satisfaction with disclosure of disability, *Developmental Medicine and Child Neurology*, 35: 816–25.

Sloper, P. and Turner, S. (1993b) Risk and resistance factors in the adaptation of parents of children with severe physical disability, *Journal of Child Psychology and Psychiatry*, 34: 167–88.

Smaje, C. (1995) *Health, Race and Ethnicity: Making Sense of the Evidence*. London: Kings Fund Institute.

Smith, J.A., Espeland, M., Bellevue, R. *et al.* (1996) Pregnancy in sickle cell disease: experience of the cooperative study of sickle cell disease, *Obstetrics and Gynecology*, 87: 199–204.

Smith, R. (1992) Using a mock trial to make a difficult clinical decision, *British Medical Journal*, 305: 1284–7.

Social Service Inspectorate (1994) *Children in Need: Report of Issues Arising from Regional Social Services Inspectorate Workshops*. London: Department of Health.

Sopher, K. (1986) *Humanism and Anti-humanism*. Hutchinson: London.

Stacey, M. (1996) The new genetics: a feminist view, in T. Marteau and M. Richards (eds) *The Troubled Helix: Social and Psychological Implications of the New Human Genetics*. Cambridge: Cambridge University Press.

Stark, L.J., Dahlquist, L.M. and Collins, F.L. (1987) Improving children's compliance with diabetes management, *Clinical Psychology Review*, 7: 223–42.

Steinberg, M.H. (1999) Management of sickle cell disease, *New England Journal of Medicine*, 340(13): 1021–30.

Stimmel, B. (1993) *Pain Analgesia and Addiction*. New York: Raven Press.

Stimson, G. and Webb, B. (1975) *Going to See the Doctor: The Consultation Process in General Practice*. London: Routledge.

Strasser, B.J. (1999) Perspectives: molecular medicine. Sickle cell anemia, a molecular disease, *Science*, 286(5444): 1488–90.

Streetly, A., Dick, M. and Layton, M. (1993) Sickle cell disease: the case for co-ordinated information, *British Medical Journal*, 306: 1491–2.

Streetly, A., Maxwell, K. and Mejia, A. (1997) *Sickle Cell Disorders in Greater London: A Needs Assessment of Screening and Care Services, The Fair Shares for London Report*. London: Department of Public Health Medicine, UMDS and St Thomas's Hospital.

Stuart, O. (1996) 'Yes, we mean black disabled people too': thoughts on community care and disabled people from black and minority ethnic communities, in W.I.U. Ahmad and K. Atkin (eds) *'Race' and Community Care*. Buckingham: Open University Press.

Sturgeon, P., Itano, H.A. and Bergren, W.R. (1955) Clinical manifestations of inherited abnormal haemoglobins. I: The interaction of hemoglobin-S with hemoglobin-D, *Blood*, 10: 389–404.

Swift, A.V., Cohen, M.J., Hynd, G.W. *et al.* (1989) Neuropsychological impairment in children with sickle cell anaemia, *Paediatrics*, 84: 1077–85.

Sydenstricker, V.P. (1924) Further observations on sickle cell anemia, *Journal of the American Medical Association*, 23: 12–15.

Sydenstricker, V.P., Mulherin, W.A. and Houseal, R.W. (1923) Sickle cell anemia: report of two cases in children with necroscopy in one case, *American Journal of Diseases in Children*, 26: 132–54.

Tapper, M. (1999) *In the Blood: Sickle Cell Anemia and the Politics of Race*. Philadelphia, PA: University of Pennsylvania Press.

Tarry, W.F., Duckett, J.W. and Snyder, H.M. (1987) Urological complications of sickle cell disease in a pediatric population, *Journal of Urology*, 138(3): 592–4.

Telfair, J. (1994) Factors in the long term adjustment of children and adolescents with sickle cell disease: conceptualizations and review of the literature, in K.B. Nash (ed.) *Psychosocial Aspects of Sickle Cell Disease: Past, Present and Future Directions of Research*. New York: The Haworth Press.

Telfair, J., Myers, J. and Drezner, S. (1994) Transfer as a component of the transition of adolescent with sickle cell disease to adult care, *Journal of Adolescent Health*, 15(7): 558–65.

Thom, D. and Jennings, M. (1996) Human pedigree and the best stock: from eugenics to genetics, in T. Marteau and M. Richards (eds) *The Troubled Helix: Social and Psychological Implications of the New Human Genetics*. Cambridge: Cambridge University Press.

Thomas, A.N., Pattison, C. and Serjeant, G.R. (1982) Causes of death in sickle-cell disease in Jamaica, *British Medical Journal*, 285: 633–5.

Thomas, E.D., Buckner, C.D. and Sanders, J.E. (1982) Marrow transplantation for thalassaemia, *Lancet*, ii: 227–9.

Thomas, V.N., Wilson-Barnet, J. and Goodhart, F. (1998) The role of cognitive-behavioural therapy in the management of pain in patients with sickle cell disease, *Journal of Advanced Nursing*, 27(5): 1002–9.

Thompson, C. (1995) Umbilical cords: turning garbage into clinical gold, *Science*, 268: 805–6.

Thompson, R.J. (1994a) Stability and change in psychological adjustments of mothers of children and adolescents with cystic fibrosis and sickle cell disease, *Journal of Paediatric Psychology*, 19(2): 171–88.

Thompson, R.J. (1994b) Psychological adjustment of a child with sickle cell disease: stability and change over a ten month period, *Journal of Consulting and Clinical Psychology*, 62(4): 856–60.

Torkington, N.P.K. (1983) *The Racial Politics of Health: A Liverpool Profile*. Liverpool: Department of Sociology, University of Liverpool.

Tozer, R. (1996) My brother's keeper? Sustaining sibling support, *Health and Social Care in the Community*, 4(3): 177–81.

Tsiantis, J., Dragonas, T., Richardson, C. *et al*. (1996) Psychosocial problems and adjustment of children with beta-thalassaemia and their families, *European Child and Adolescent Psychiatry*, 5: 193–203.

Turner, B. (1989) From orientalism to globalism, *Sociology*, 24(4): 629–38.

Turner, S. and Sloper, P. (1992) Paediatricians' practice in disclosure and follow-up of severe physical disability in young children, *Developmental Medicine and Child Neurology*, 34: 348–58.

Twigg, J. (1997) Deconstructing the social bath: help with bathing at home for older and disabled people, *Journal of Social Policy*, 26(2): 211–32.

Twigg, J. and Atkin, K. (1994) *Carers Perceived: Policy and Practice in Informal Care*. Buckingham: Open University Press.

Vellodi, A., Picton, S., Downie, C.J. *et al*. (1994) Bone marrow transplantation for thalassaemia: experience of two British centres, *Bone Marrow Transplantation*, 13(5): 559–62.

Vermylen, C.H., Cornu, G., Philippe, J. *et al*. (1991) Bone marrow transplant in sickle cell anaemia, *Archives of Disease in Childhood*, 66: 1195–8.

Vichinsky, E., Hurst, D., Earles, A., Kleman, K. and Lubin, B. (1988) Newborn screening for sickle cell disease: effect on mortality, *Paediatrics*, 81: 749–55.

Vichinsky, E.P., Johnson, R.J. and Lubin, B.H. (1982) Multidisciplinary approach to pain management in sickle cell disease, *American Journal of Pediatric Hematology/Oncology*, 4: 328–33.

Vichinsky, E.P., Styles, L.A., Colangelo, L.H. *et al.* (1997) Acute chest syndrome in sickle cell disease: clinical presentation and course, *Blood*, 89: 1787–92.

Vlachou, A. (1997) *Struggles for Inclusive Education: An Ethnographic Study*. Buckingham: Open University Press.

Vullo, R., Modell, B. and Georganda, E. (1995) *What is Thalassaemia?* Cyprus: The Thalassaemia International Federation.

Wainscoat, J.S., Thein, S.L. and Weatherall, D.J. (1987) Thalassaemia intermedia, *Blood Reviews*, 1(4): 273–9.

Walco, G.A. and Dampier, C.D. (1990) Pain in children and adolescents with sickle cell disease: a descriptive study, *Journal of Paediatric Psychology*, 15(5): 643.

Waldrop, R.D. and Mandry, C. (1995) Health professional perceptions of opioid dependence among patients with pain, *American Journal of Emergency Medicine*, 13: 529–31.

Walker, R. and Ahmad, W.I.U. (1994) Windows of opportunity in rotting frames: care providers' perspectives on community care and black communities, *Critical Social Policy*, 40: 46–68.

Walters, M.C., Patience, M., Leisenring, W. *et al.* (1996) Bone marrow transplantation for sickle cell disease, *New England Journal of Medicine*, 335(6): 369–428.

Wang, C.H. and Schilling, R.F. (1995) Myocardial infarction and thalassemia trait: an example of heterozygote advantage, *American Journal of Hematology*, 49(1): 73–5.

Ward, S.J., Simini, B., Meltzer, B.A. *et al.* (1996) Correspondence re sickle cell pain crisis, *Lancet*, 347: 261–3.

Ware, R.E., Zimmerman, S.A. and Schultz, W.H. (1999) Hydroxurea as an alternative to blood transfusions for the prevention of recurrent stroke in children with sickle cell disease, *Blood*, 94(9): 3022–66.

Washburn, R.E. (1911) Peculiar elongated and sickle shaped red blood corpuscles in a case of severe anemia, *Virginia Medicine*, 15: 490–3.

Watson, E.K., Mayall, E.S., Lamb, J., Chapple, J. and Williamson, B. (1992) Psychological and social consequences of community carrier screening programme for cystic fibrosis, *Lancet*, 340(8813): 217–20.

Weatherall, D.J. (1993) The treatment of thalassemia: slow progress and new dilemmas, *New England Journal of Medicine*, 329: 877–9.

Weatherall, D.J. (1996) Thalassaemia: a global public health problem, *Nature Medicine*, 2(8): 847–9.

Weatherall, D.J. (1997a) ABC of clinical haematology: the hereditary anaemias, *British Medical Journal*, 314: 492–6.

Weatherall, D.J. (1997b) Fortnightly review: the thalassaemia, *British Medical Journal*, 314(7095): 1675–8.

Weatherall, D.J. (1999) Thalassemia and malaria: new insights into an old problem, *Proceedings of the Association of American Physicians*, 111(4): 278–82.

Weatherall, D.J. (2000) Single gene disorders or complex traits: lessons from the thalassaemias and other monogenic diseases, *British Medical Journal*, 321: 1117–20.

Weatherall, D.J. and Clegg, J. (1981) *The Thalassaemia Syndromes*. Oxford: Blackwell Scientific.

Weiss, J.O. (1992) Support groups for patients with genetic disorders and their families, *Paediatric Clinics of America*, 39(1): 13–23.

Wertz, D.C., Sorenson, J.R. and Heeren, T.C. (1986) Client's interpretations of risks provided in genetic counselling, *American Journal of Human Genetics*, 39(2): 253–64.

Wertz, D., Fletcher, J.C. and Mulvihill, J.J. (1990) Medical geneticists confront ethical dilemmas: cross cultural comparisons among 18 nations, *American Journal of Human Genetics*, 46: 1200–13.

Whipple, G.H. and Bradford, W.L. (1936) Mediterranean disease – thalassaemia (erythroblastic anaemia of Cooley): associated pigment abnormalities simulating hemochromatosis, *Journal of Paediatrics*, 9: 279.

Whitten, C.F. (1973) *Informing the Public, Approaches, Problems and Solutions*. New York: Harlem Hospital Comprehensive Sickle Cell Center.

Whitten, C.F. and Fischoff, J. (1974) Psychosocial effects of sickle cell disease, *Archives of Internal Medicine*, 133: 681–9.

Williams, F. (1996) Race, welfare and community care: a historical perspective, in W.I.U. Ahmad and K. Atkin (eds) *'Race' and Community Care*. Buckingham: Open University Press.

Williams, G. (1984) The genesis of chronic illness: narrative reconstruction, *Sociology of Health and Illness*, 6: 175–200.

Williams, R. (1993) Religion and illness, in A. Radley (ed.) *Worlds of Illness: Biographical and Cultural Perspectives on Health and Disease*. London: Routledge.

Wilson, J.B., Headlee, M.E. and Huisman, T.H.J. (1983) A new high performance liquid chromatographic procedure for the separation and quantitation of various hemoglobins in adults and newborns, *Journal of Laboratory and Clinical Medicine*, 10: 174–86.

Wjst, M., Roell, G., Dold, S. *et al.* (1996) Psychosocial characteristics of asthma, *Journal of Clinical Epidemiology*, 49(4): 461–6.

Wolman, I.J. (1964) Transfusion therapy in Cooley's anemia: growth and health as related to long range hemoglobin levels: a progress report, *Annals of the New York Academy of Sciences*, 119: 736–47.

Wong, W.Y., Powars, D.R., Chan, L. *et al.* (1992) Polysaccharide encapsulated bacterial infection in sickle cell anemia: a thirty year experience, *American Journal of Haematology*, 39: 176–82.

Wonke, B., Telfer, P., Garson, J.A. and Hoffbrand, A.V. (1996) Alpha interferon alone and in combination with Ribavirin for hepatitis C virus (HCV) in multiply transfused thalassaemic patients, *Thalassaemia International Federation News*, 18: 16.

Wood, P. (1980) The language of disablement: a glossary relating to disease and its consequences, *International Rehabilitation Medicine*, 2: 86–92.

World Health Organization (1983) Community control of the hereditary anaemias: memorandum from a WHO meeting, *Bulletin of the World Health Organization*, 61: 63–80.

World Health Organization (1988) *The Haemoglobinopathies in Europe: A Combined Report on Two WHO Meetings*, Copenhagen: World Health Organization Regional Office.

World Health Organization (1994) *Guidelines for the Control of Haemoglobin Disorders*. Geneva: World Health Organization Hereditary Diseases Programme.

Yardumian, A. (1993) The north Middlesex hospital experience of pain control, in J. Shankleman and A. May (eds) *Pain in Sickle Cell Disease: Setting Standards of*

Care. (The proceedings of a one-day conference held on 19 September 1991, in the University of Wales College of Medicine, Cardiff on behalf of The Sickle and Thalassaemia Association of Counsellors.) Cardiff: Community Health Unit, South Glamorgan Health Authority.

Yardumian, A., Olujohungbe, A. and Cinkotai, K. (1999) Register cannot replace prospective studies in sickle cell disease, *British Medical Journal*, 318(7184): 671–2.

Younge, P. (1990) £175,000 for ruined life, *The Voice*, 405: 1–3.

Zani, B., Dipalma, A. and Vullo, C. (1995) Psychosocial aspects of chronic illness in adolescents with thalassemia major, *Journal of Adolescence*, 18(4): 387–402.

Zeuner, D., Ades, E.A., Karnon, J. *et al.* (1999) *Antenatal and Neonatal Haemoglobinopathy Screening in the UK: Review and Economic Analysis.* Health Technology Assessment Report, 3(11).

Zola, I.K. (1975) Medicine as an institution of social control, in G. Cox and A.A. Mead (eds) *Sociology of Medical Practice.* London: Macmillan.

Zurlo, M.G., De Stefano, P. and Borgna-Pignatti, C. (1989) Survival and causes of death in thalassemia major, *Lancet*, 2: 27–30.

Index